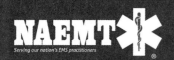

Serving our nation's EMS practitioners

SECOND EDITION

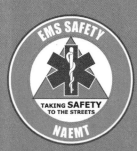

EMS Safety

EMS Safety Committee of the National Association of Emergency Medical Technicians

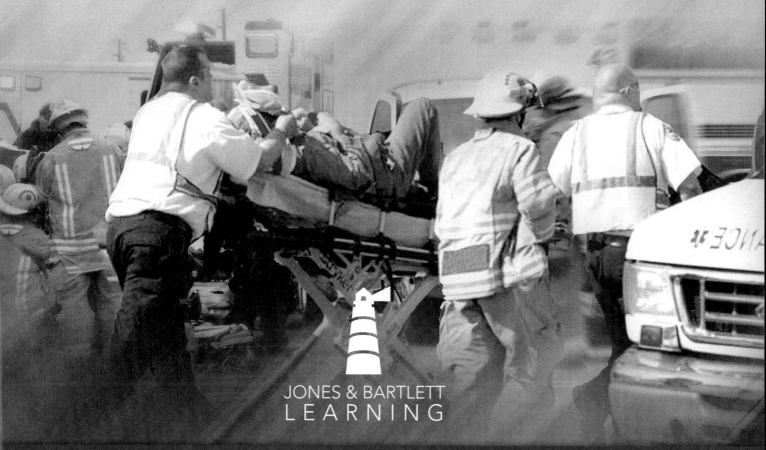

JONES & BARTLETT
LEARNING

World Headquarters
Jones & Bartlett Learning
5 Wall Street
Burlington, MA 01803
978-443-5000
info@jblearning.com
www.jblearning.com

Jones & Bartlett Learning books and products are available through most bookstores and online booksellers. To contact Jones & Bartlett Learning directly, call 800-832-0034, fax 978-443-8000, or visit our website, www.jblearning.com.

10127-0

Production Credits
VP, Executive Publisher: Kimberly Brophy
Executive Editor—EMS: Christine Emerton
Senior Content Developer: Jennifer Deforge-Kling
Associate Director of Production: Jenny L. Corriveau
VP, Sales—Public Safety Group: Matthew Maniscalco
Director of Sales, Public Safety Group: Patricia Einstein
VP, Marketing: Alisha Weisman
VP, Manufacturing and Inventory Control: Therese Connell

Manufacturing and Inventory Control Supervisor: Amy Bacus
Composition: diacriTech
Cover Design: Kristin E. Parker
Rights & Media Specialist: Robert Boder
Cover Image: Courtesy of Sunstar Paramedics. Photographed by Greg Moran.
Printing and Binding: RR Donnelley
Cover Printing: RR Donnelley

Library of Congress Cataloging-in-Publication Data
EMS safety/National Association of Emergency Medical Technicians. – Second edition.
    pages cm
    Includes index.
    ISBN 978-1-284-04111-8 (pbk.)
1. Emergency medical services. 2. Emergency medical technicians. I. National Association of Emergency Medical Technicians (U.S.)
    RA645.5.E455 2015
    362.18--dc23

2015023000

6048
Printed in the United States of America
19 18 17 16   10 9 8 7 6 5 4 3 2

BRIEF CONTENTS

CHAPTER 1 Taking Safety to the Streets 1

CHAPTER 2 Crew Resource Management 9

CHAPTER 3 Emergency Vehicle Safety 25

CHAPTER 4 Responsibilities in Roadway Operations 41

CHAPTER 5 Patient Handling 51

CHAPTER 6 Patient, Practitioner, and Bystander Safety 67

CHAPTER 7 Personal Health 83

CHAPTER 8 Conclusion 95

APPENDIX A Scene Safety for Infectious Diseases 101

GLOSSARY 109

INDEX 111

CONTENTS

CHAPTER 1 **Taking Safety to the Streets** **1**

Introduction 2
A Dangerous Job 3
    Overview 3
    Motor Vehicle Crashes. 3
    Breaking Down the Risks 4
Identifying the Risks. 5
    From the Top Down. 5
    Personal Responsibility 5
A Change in Culture. 5
    Healthy Communication 5
    From the Top Down. 6
    The Bottom Line 6

CHAPTER 2 **Crew Resource Management** **9**

Introduction 10
Crew Resource Management. 10
    CRM Components 10
    Incident Command System 11
Teamwork 13
    Conflict and Respect 13
Leaders 13
Situational Awareness 14
Open Communications. 17
    Inquiry 17
    Advocacy 18
    Conflict Resolution 18
    Decision 19
    Observe and Critique. 19
    Discuss Options 19
Decision Making. 20
Reducing Human Error. 20
    Errors Are Not Random. 20
    Risk Assessment 20
    Personal Strategies 21
    Postincident Analysis (PIA) 21

CHAPTER 3 **Emergency Vehicle Safety** **25**

Introduction 26
Avoiding Collisions. 26
    What the Data Say. 27
    Personal Experience. 28
    Risk Factors. 28

Backing. 30
Rate of Closure 31
Speed 31
Total Stopping Distance. 31
Emergency Driving 32
Distractions. 32
Text Messaging 33
Codriving. 33
Distracted Driving. 34
Habits Need to Change 34
Vehicle Inspections and Maintenance. 34
Vehicle Inspections 34
Vehicle Maintenance. 34
Respect Your Vehicles 35
Everyone and Everything Restrained 35
Seat Belt Use 35
Patient Compartment 35
Risk Mitigation 36
Avoid Injury 36
Working in Motion. 36
Preparation and Ergonomics Actions 36
Helmets 37
Transporting Patients. 37
Adults. 37
Pediatric Challenges 37

CHAPTER 4 Responsibilities in Roadway Operations 41
Introduction 42
The Dangers of the Road. 42
Preplanning for Safety. 43
Traffic Incident Management Plans 43
Vehicle Visibility. 43
Arrival and Scene Size-Up 44
Operations 46
Emergency Lighting. 46
Air Ambulance. 47

CHAPTER 5 Patient Handling. 51
Introduction 52
Safe Patient Movement. 52
Safety Begins with You 53
Unsafe Patient Handling: Physical and Psychological Harm to Patients. 53
Pediatric Patients. 53
Bariatric Patients 53
Geriatric Patients. 54
Unsafe Patient Handling: Physical and Psychological Harm to EMS Practitioners. 54
The Risks and Consequences of Back Injury. 54
Patient Handling 55
Behavioral Controls. 57
Evaluation of the Patient and Environment. 57
Patient Assessment. 57
Environmental Assessment 58
Form a Lifting and Moving Plan 59
Question 1: Environment 59
Question 2: Patient 59
Question 3: Personnel Preparation. 59
Question 4: Equipment 61
Equipment Maintenance 64

CHAPTER 6   Patient, Practitioner, and Bystander Safety 67

Introduction 68
Personal Safety 68
Crime Scenes 68
    The Hazards of Illegal Drugs 69
    The Hazards of Alcohol 69
    Active Shooter Incidents 69
Secure Facilities 70
Communication Skills during Times of Stress 71
Violence against EMS Practitioners 72
    The Six Ds 72
    Patient or Potential Attacker? 73
    Violent Encounters 74
Weapons 74
Excited Delirium Syndrome 75
Restraining a Patient 76
    Restraint Pitfalls 76
Errors in Patient Care 76
    Medication Errors 77
    Patient Falls 77
    Delays in Treatment 77
    Equipment Failures 78
    Infections 78

CHAPTER 7   Personal Health 83

Introduction 84
Mental Health 84
    Depression 85
    Anxiety 85
Resiliency 85
    Why Is Resiliency Important? 86
    How Do We Address the Problem? 86
    What's in the Resiliency Toolbox? 86
Fitness and Health 89
    Exercise Guidelines 89
    A Healthy Diet 90

CHAPTER 8   Conclusion 95

Introduction 96
Significant Steps in Creating an EMS Culture of Safety 97
    Ambulance 97
    NAEMT 98
    EMS Safety Foundation 98
    Federal Regulations 98
    International Association of Fire Chiefs 98
EMS Culture of Safety 98
    Safety Begins with You 98

APPENDIX A   Scene Safety for Infectious Diseases 101

GLOSSARY 109

INDEX 111

Contributors

EMS Safety Committee

Michael Szczygiel, BS
Committee Chair and Lead Editor
Senior Loss Control Specialist, Medical Transportation
Markel Specialty Programs
Overland Park, Kansas

Taz Meyer, BS, EMT-P
Committee Co-Chair
Chief Executive Officer
St. Charles County Ambulance District
St. Peters, Missouri

Peter Dworsky, MPH, NRP, CBRM
Corporate Director of Support Services
MONOC-Mobile Health Services
Neptune, New Jersey

Jason Schiederer, MS, NRP
EMS Educator
Indianapolis, Indiana
EPIC Implementation Director of Training
Eskenazi Health
Indianapolis, Indiana

Paul Hinchey, MD
Medical Director for the EMS Safety Committee
President of East Coast Operations
Evolution Health
Dallas, Texas

Charlene Cobb, NRP
Community Outreach Coordinator
Sunstar Paramedics
Largo, Florida

Rob Garrett, MS, ASP, NRP
Regional Safety & Risk Manager
AMR
Greenwood Village, Colorado

Subject Matter Experts

Philip Callahan, Ph.D., EMT-P
Veterans' Education College of Agricultural and Life Sciences
Emeritus University of Arizona
Tucson, Arizona

Jeff T. Dyar, NRP, BS
Fire Commissioner and President of the Board
Upper Pine Fire Protection District
Bayfield, Colorado

Bryan Fass, ATC, LAT, CSCS, EMT-P (retired)
Fass Consulting LLC
Charlotte, North Carolina

Bill Coll
Infection Preventionist
Office of the Medical Director
Austin-Travis County EMS
Austin, Texas

Bruce Evans, MPA, NRP
Fire Chief
Upper Pine River Fire Protection District
Bayfield, Colorado

Mike Grill, MS, NRP
EMS Regional Program Director
Centura Health South Denver EMS Team
Denver, Colorado

Paul LeSage, FF, EMT-P, AS, BA, CFM
Assistant Chief (retired)
Portland, Oregon

Michael Wm. Marks, Ph.D., ABPP
Lead Psychologist
Assistant Clinical Professor, University of Arizona
SAVAHCS
Tucson, Arizona

Scott Sholes, BA, NRP
EMS Chief
Durango Fire & Rescue
Durango, Colorado

Glenn Luedtke, NRP
Former Chairman, Director (retired)
Sussex County EMS
Adjunct Assistant Professor
Emergency Health Services Program
The George Washington University School of Medicine and
Health Science
Washington D.C.

Michael Shelton, NRP
Driver Instructor
MedStar
Burleson, Texas

Kip Teitsort, EMT-P
Founder
DT4EMS, LLC
Cartersville, Georgia

National Association of Emergency Medical Technicians 2015 Board of Directors

Officers

President: Chuck Kearns
President-Elect: Dennis Rowe
Immediate Past President: Don Lundy
Secretary: Bruce Evans
Treasurer: Scott Matin
Medical Director: Paul Hinchey, MD

Directors

Sean Britton   Jason Scheiderer
Robert Luckritz   Terry David
Chad McIntyre   Troy Tuke
Cory Richter   Ben Chlapek
Aimee Binning   Matt Zavadsky

Reviewers

Katrina Altenhofen, MPH, Paramedic
Child Passenger Safety Seat Technician Instructor
National Association of State EMS Officials-Pediatric Emergency
Care Council
Department of Transportation-National EMS Advisory Council
Washington, Iowa

Brian K. Andrews, NRP
County Ambulance Service
Pittsfield, Massachusetts

Daniel Armstrong, DPT, EMT
Queensborough Community College
Bayside, New York

Bruce Barry, RN, CEN, CPEN, NRP
Peak Paramedicine, LLC
Wilmington, New York

David Burdett, NR-P
Hamilton County EMS
Chattanooga, Tennessee

Kristopher Ambrosia, NCEE, FF/Paramedic
Morton, Illinois

Paul Arens, B.S., NRP
Iowa Central Community College
Fort Dodge, Iowa

Michael Baker, US Army Retired, NRP
Save A Life San Antonio
Converse, Texas

Trent R. Brass, MPH, RRT, EMT-P
SwedishAmerican Health System
Rockford, Illinois

Lance Corey, Paramedic, I/C
Oceana County EMS
Hart, Michigan

Matthew Dick, EMT-P, EMSI, PSSI
Delaware Area Career Center
Delaware, Ohio

Rom Duckworth, LP
New England Center for Rescue & Emergency Medicine
Sherman, Connecticut

Dan Evans, EMT, CIC
LaGuardia Community College/CUNY
Long Island City, New York

Scott A. Gano, BS, NRP, FP-C, CCEMT-P
Assistant Professor
Paramedic Program Director
Columbus State Community College
Columbus, Ohio

John Gosford, MS, NRP
College of Southern Maryland
Waldorf, Maryland

Lt. Kathleen D. Grote, NRP
Anne Arundel County Fire Department
Millersville, Maryland

Janelle Johnson, Paramedic/Instructor
Metropolitan EMS of Little Rock
Little Rock, Arkansas

Steven M. Kirschbaum, Paramedic
SwedishAmerican Health System
Rockford, Illinois

Sarah Leach, BS, LP, NRP, CCEMTP
North Blanco County EMS
Johnson City, Texas

Jane E. MacArthur, MS, NRP, I/C
StarFire EMS, Emergency Medical Educators
Winchester, Massachusetts

Scott A. Matin, MBA, NRP
MONOC Mobile Health Services
Wall, New Jersey

Janice McKay, RN, CEN, CFRN, VAEMT-B
Nightingale Regional Air Ambulance
Norfolk, Virginia

Daniel W. Murdock, BT, NRP, CIC
SUNY Cobleskill Paramedic Program
Cobleskill, New York

James Dinsch, PhD(c), NRP, CCEMTP
Indian River State College
Fort Pierce, Florida

Michael J. Dunaway, BHS, NRP, CCP, NCEE
Greenville Technical College EMT Department
Lyman, South Carolina

Michael Frith, MS, LP, NCEE
Paramedics Plus
San Leandro, California

Doug Gernerd, NRP
George E. Moerkirk Emergency Medical Institute
Allentown, Pennsylvania

Shane Grier, NRP, NCOEMS Level I
Chocowinity EMS
Chocowinity, North Carolina

Scott A. Jaeggi, BA, EMT-P
Rio Hondo College Fire Academy
Santa Fe Springs, California

Richard Kaufman, MBA, NRP
EMS Institute
Pittsburgh, Pennsylvania

Greg LaMay, NRP, NCEE
East Texas Medical Center EMS
Tyler, Texas

Michael E. Lisa, BS, NJ EMT-Instructor
Trinitas Medical Center
Elizabeth, New Jersey

Susan M Macklin, BS, EMT-P
Central Carolina Community College
Sanford, North Carolina

Donna McHenry, MS, NRP
Los Alamos Fire Department
Los Alamos, New Mexico

Steven Mountfort, CCEMT-P, NCEE
Florida Hospital EMS
Orlando, Florida

Jodi Mannino Nevandro, RN, MSN, PhD
Santa Monica Fire Department
Santa Monica, California

Amiel B. Oliva, BSN, RN, REMT-I
Emergency Medical Responder Healthcare and
Safety Institute
Quezon City, Philippines

Lt. Guy Peifer, Paramedic
Yonkers Fire Department
New York, New York

Jared C. Schoenfeld, CCEMT-P, NRP
Haywood Community College
Waynesville, North Carolina

Chris Ottolini, EMT-P, CPT
Paramedic Supervisor
Adjunct Instructor
Coast Life Support District
Gualala, California
Santa Rosa Junior College Public Safety Training Center
Windsor, California

Mark Podgwaite, Sr., NRAEMT, NECEMS, I/C
Vermont EMS District 5
Northfield, Vermont

John B. Walker, BS, EMT-P
Norfolk Fire-Rescue
Norfolk, Virginia

CHAPTER 1

© Barbol/Shutterstock

Taking Safety to the Streets

CHAPTER OBJECTIVES

After reading this chapter, the participant will be able to:

- Describe the unsafe aspects of working in emergency medical services (EMS)

- Describe how to identify the potential hazards in daily activities

- Describe the cultural changes required to make EMS safer

© Barbol/Shutterstock

SCENARIO

On your way into work, you notice that traffic is becoming congested, and you realize you're going to be late. As you're pulling into the station, you see that your partner also is just pulling in. You're both 15 minutes late. Both of you quickly grab your gear and toss it in the ambulance as the tones go off. There has been no time to check your ambulance, nor receive a hand-off from the off-going crew.

Dispatch reports that a 61-year-old male is in cardiac arrest. On arrival, your partner opens the side cabinet to retrieve the cardiac monitor and realizes it's not there. You look in the back of the unit and notice that your first-in bag is missing the intubation equipment.

1. How could this have been mitigated from the start?
2. What is your first priority in this situation?
3. What actions are required next?

Introduction

Emergency medical services (EMS) is a profession of extremes. One moment, we are dealing with patient care situations that stress our cognitive and psychomotor skills in potentially life-threatening environments. In the next moment, we are performing a routine patient transport. We leap from emotionally charged scenes to emotionally neutral ones, often without the opportunity for physical or mental recovery **FIGURE 1-1**. The transition from an intense situation to a calm one can be exhausting and lead us to let down our guard during the moments of calm. After running "hot" during a call, we may be less attentive to traffic while driving back to the station after a call.

The constant cycle of crisis and calm may lead us to pay less attention to our surroundings and subsequently fail to process sensorimotor cues in the environment. **Sensorimotor cues** are the sights, sounds, and smells that create an awareness of environmental conditions; this awareness may prompt a behavioral response. For example, the smell of smoke could prompt you to look for a fire.

EMS practitioners and patients are not harmed only in overtly dangerous situations, such as driving in an ice storm. A growing number of patients are injured, sometimes critically, in nonemergent patient handling events, such as moving a patient from a bed to a stretcher. When a task seems "routine," there is a risk of the mind slipping into **complacency**,

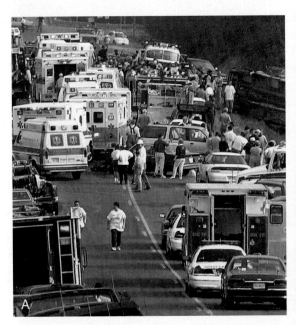
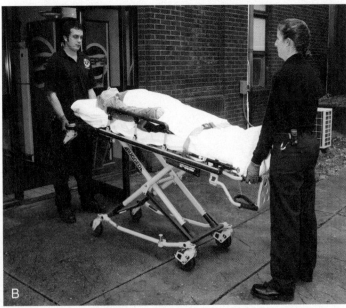

Figure 1-1   EMS is a profession of extremes. **A**. One moment, you may be dealing with a life-threatening situation. **B**. The next moment, you may be moving a patient.

© David Crigger, Bristol Herald Courier/AP Images; © Jones & Bartlett Learning.

which occurs when you believe you are so good at your job that you stop thinking about how to do it properly. When you stop thinking about your job, you lose the ability to maintain situational awareness.

You may be thinking that you have taken driving courses and patient handling training and have participated in a variety of other safety-oriented activities. You have onboard monitoring equipment and power cots. You use all the appropriate personal protective equipment on every call. You know the dangers of intersections, the use of lights and sirens, and the plague of distracted drivers. What else can you possibly do to improve your safety? *EMS Safety* will explore the preventative measures that you and your colleagues can take to improve personal, patient, and bystander safety.

Safety is a dynamic issue that changes from moment to moment. Weather, traffic flow, and bystanders becoming unruly all alter scene safety. Remember the concept of homeostasis from your initial training? Cells constantly engage in a variety of actions to maintain a balanced internal environment. Homeostatic mechanisms work to limit the damage that cells incur when assaulted by everything from hypoxia to mechanical forces. Likewise, EMS practitioners need to develop a set of homeostatic mechanisms—or behaviors—to constantly adapt to the ever-changing environment and limit the potential risks to ourselves, our patients, and bystanders. *EMS Safety* will teach you how to develop ingrained behaviors that will allow you to adapt naturally to the current situation and address issues before they become threats. Proactive prevention is the key to maintaining your safety and the safety of your partner, patients, and bystanders.

STAY IN THE FIELD

The purpose of *EMS Safety* is to change the culture of safety in the EMS profession and in each organization. The key to changing the culture is understanding and mitigating the perceived risk. This change will occur only if EMS practitioners and agency management embrace the importance of applying safety practices and understanding risk.

A Dangerous Job

Overview

EMS is a dangerous job for both professional and volunteer EMS practitioners. Compared with other professions:

- The fatality rate for EMS practitioners is *2 ½ times* the national average[1] TABLES 1-1 and 1-2.
- EMS practitioners are *3 times more likely* than the average worker to miss work as result of injury.[2]

Table 1-1 Transportation-Related Fatalities

	Transportation-Related Fatalities (per 100,000)
National Average	2.0
Fire Fighters	5.7
Police Officers	6.1
EMS Practitioners	9.6

Data from: Kahn CA. EMS, first responders, and crash injury. *Top Emerg Med*. 2006;26:68–74.

Table 1-2 Fatal Occupational Injuries

	Fatal Occupational Injuries (per 100,000)
National Average	5.0
Fire Fighters	16.5
Police Officers	14.2
EMS Practitioners	12.7

Data from: Maguire BJ, Hunting KL, Smith GS, Levick NR. Occupational fatalities in emergency medical services: a hidden crisis. *Ann Emer Med*. 2002;40:625–632.

Motor Vehicle Crashes

According to the National Highway Traffic Safety Administration (NHTSA), between 1992 and 2011, there were 4,500 accidents involving ambulances, for an average of about 12 motor vehicle crashes (MVCs) involving ambulances a day FIGURE 1-2. Of those accidents, 65% resulted in property damage, 34% resulted in injuries, and less than 1% resulted in fatalities. The breakdown of those fatalities:

- Ambulance driver – 4%
- Ambulance passenger – 21%
- Occupants of another vehicle – 63%
- Nonoccupants – 12%

Of the 34% who were injured:

- Ambulance driver – 17%
- Ambulance passenger – 29%
- Occupants of another vehicle – 54%

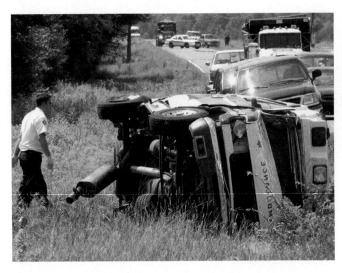

Figure 1-2   According to the NHTSA, between 1992 and 2011, there was an average of about 12 MVCs involving ambulances a day.

© Gary Lloyd, The Decatur Daily/AP Photos

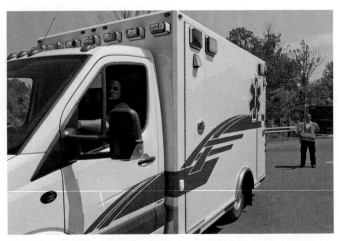

Figure 1-3   Because of the dangers inherent in operating in reverse, many agencies have policies, such as using a spotter, to help the emergency vehicle operator back safely.

© Jones & Bartlett Learning. Photographed by Glen E. Ellman.

The statistics show that in MVCs involving ambulance crashes, the ambulance driver is less likely to be killed or injured than ambulance passengers, occupants of other vehicles, and nonoccupants. This means that the person responsible for driving the ambulance safely carries the least amount of personal risk during an MVC. The presence of a moving ambulance should not be a hazard to the general public, and the general public should not become "collateral damage" because of an MVC with an ambulance.

In MVCs involving ambulances, 58% of accidents were lights-and-sirens events, and 42% were nonemergent driving events. Clearly, nonemergent driving events pose an almost equal risk of an MVC as lights-and-sirens events. This is one reason it is critical to be aware of potential safety hazards and be proactive at all times.

In most states, running with lights and sirens allows ambulance drivers to exceed the posted speed limit and disregard usual driving restrictions while practicing due regard for the general public. When MVCs occur at high speeds, the force of the colliding objects increases, and the risk of traumatic injury to the vehicle occupants also increases. The risk of lights-and-sirens events is readily apparent.

Nonemergent driving events clearly pose a risk, too. One of the biggest risks when driving nonemergent is operating in reverse and backing. Many agencies have policies regarding backing or teach proper backing techniques **FIGURE 1-3** . Although education will help to mitigate the risk, the policy will do nothing for mitigating risk. An equal level of awareness and intensity must be applied to nonemergency and emergency driving events.

Breaking Down the Risks

EMS is a young profession with a safety culture that often overlooks real risks to our personal health and wellness. During a call, the focus of the EMS practitioner is on the rapid assessment, management, treatment, and transport of the patient. This

IN THE FIELD

Limitations to data acquisition and variations in methodologies can make statistical comparisons confusing. The NHTSA published the following limitations of their analysis of MVCs involving ambulances:

- NHTSA only includes motor vehicle crashes on public roads.
- Not all motor vehicle crashes are reported to the police.
- Ambulances may not be included on the police crash report.
- NHTSA does not identify the type of ambulance (modular vs. van) involved in the MVC.
- NHTSA does not specify where occupants are in the ambulance.

sense of urgency can be consuming, and sensorimotor cues of scene dangers may be missed. You could miss the arrival of hostile bystanders, the leak of toxic materials, or changes in the weather.

In addition, shift work, long hours, and the resulting fatigue can increase the chance of personal injury or illness. In busy EMS systems, the opportunity for adequate hydration, nutrition, rest, and stress relief can be limited.

Although Occupational Safety & Health Administration (OSHA) investigates workplace injuries and deaths, we do not yet have a mandatory database to record information on near-misses. However, we know that any of the following can put us at risk:

- Not using the proper level of personal protective equipment (PPE)
- Lack of seat belt use by ambulance occupants
- Navigating intersections
- Use of lights and sirens
- Distracted driving by both ambulance drivers and the general public

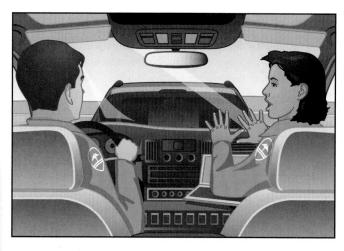

Figure 1-4 If you are riding with an emergency vehicle operator who is driving unsafely, speak up—don't sit in silence.
© Jones & Bartlett Learning.

> ### STAY IN THE FIELD
>
> More EMS practitioners than police and fire personnel die in transportation-related fatalities. Chapter 3: *Emergency Vehicle Safety* discusses how to minimize the risks to you, your partner, your patient, and the general public during transport.

Identifying the Risks
From the Top Down

Identification and mitigation of risk begin at the top and are the responsibility of every member of the agency. With the knowledge that the majority of risks associated with EMS involve MVCs and patient-handling events, prospective employees should be evaluated closely from a psychological and physical perspective. The driving records of potential employees should be screened and criminal background checks performed. Keeping the ambulance keys out of the hands of a proven reckless driver will protect the agency, EMS practitioners, patients, and the general public. Ideally, psychological testing would also be performed to assess for tendencies toward engaging in reckless behaviors. Because of the physical requirements of the job, physical readiness should also be determined through validated testing such as the Candidate Physical Agility Test (CPAT) or another reliable, validated physical ability test.

The agency should communicate a clear baseline level of behavioral expectations among EMS practitioners. Behaviors that fall outside of these stated expectations should be identified and corrected immediately. For example, an EMS practitioner riding with an emergency vehicle operator who is driving unsafely should speak up and tell the driver to correct the behavior **FIGURE 1-4**. If the behavior continues or is repeated, superiors must be informed.

Personal Responsibility

EMS practitioners must use common sense, critical thinking, and situational awareness. It is unrealistic to expect that an agency will craft policies and procedures to address every potential risk in the field. Is a policy needed to tell ambulance drivers to drive more slowly on ice? Is a policy needed to warn EMS practitioners to step carefully when transporting a patient down a flight of stairs? Just as it is the agency's responsibility to communicate a clear expectation that all EMS practitioners must not take unnecessary risks, EMS practitioners must *think* about what they are doing. They must determine the steps involved in a task and make certain that the task can be completed in a manner that minimizes injury to the patient, fellow EMS practitioners, and bystanders while always being aware of the constantly evolving scene.

A Change in Culture
Healthy Communication

EMS practitioners must strive to achieve "a sound mind in a healthy body," which will allow each EMS practitioner to function at his or her capacity. Personal fitness must be accompanied by social fitness. EMS practitioners must be polite and pleasant to everyone because treating others with respect is a cornerstone of good communication.

To practice proactive accident prevention, everyone needs to be aware of the potential hazards. The effectiveness of situational awareness is amplified when EMS practitioners communicate their findings with each other. However, this will not occur if interpersonal barriers exist.

> ### IN THE FIELD
>
> EMS practitioners should have a strong desire to protect each other.

From the Top Down

There should be no administrative barriers to solving safety issues. Those who report a problem should not be identified by coworkers or supervisors as contributing to a problem. The manner in which a problem will be solved and the timeline for the execution of the solution should be shared with everyone in the agency. The inability to completely fix a problem should be shared as well.

The Bottom Line

The health, well-being, and safety of EMS practitioners must be recognized as essential by employers, the public, and the EMS practitioners themselves. EMS practitioners have the right and the responsibility to insist on a safe work environment.

WRAP-UP

Summary

- The constant cycle of crisis and calm may lead EMS practitioners to pay less attention to their surroundings and subsequently fail to process sensorimotor cues in the environment.
- EMS practitioners and patients can be harmed in situations that range from the overtly dangerous, such as driving in an ice storm, to nonemergent patient handling events, such as moving a patient from a bed to a stretcher.
- When a task seems routine, there is a risk of the mind slipping into complacency. When we stop thinking about the job at hand, we lose the ability to maintain situational awareness.
- Safety is a dynamic issue that changes from moment to moment. EMS practitioners need to develop a set of ingrained behaviors to constantly adapt to the ever-changing environment and limit the potential risks to ourselves, our patients, and bystanders.
- Proactive prevention is the key to maintaining our safety and the safety of our crews, patients, and bystanders.
- EMS is a dangerous job for both professional and volunteer EMS practitioners. The statistics speak for themselves. The fatality rate for EMS practitioners is 2 ½ times the national average.[1] EMS practitioners are 3 times more likely than average workers to miss work as a result of injury.[2]
- Driving carries a significant amount of risk. According to the NHTSA, between 1992 and 2011, an average of about 12 MVCs involving ambulances occurred a day.

- In addition to the risks of the road, operating in reverse and backing pose risks to the ambulance, the ambulance crew, and bystanders. There must be an equal level of awareness and focus given to operating nonemergently and to driving with lights and sirens on.
- EMS is a young profession with a safety culture that often overlooks real risks to our personal health and wellness. During a call, our focus is on the rapid assessment, management, treatment, and transport of the patient. This sense of urgency can be consuming, and sensorimotor cues of scene dangers may be missed.
- Identification and mitigation of risk begin at the top and are the responsibility of every member of the agency.
- The agency should communicate a clear baseline level of behavioral expectations among EMS practitioners. Behaviors that fall outside these stated expectations should be identified and corrected immediately.
- EMS practitioners must use common sense, critical thinking, and situational awareness. It is unrealistic to expect that an agency will craft policies and procedures to address every potential risk in the field.
- EMS practitioners must strive to achieve "a sound mind in a healthy body," which will allow each EMS practitioner to function at his or her optimal capacity.
- EMS practitioners must be polite and pleasant to everyone because treating others with respect is a cornerstone of good communication.
- EMS practitioners have the right and the responsibility to insist on a safe work environment.

WRAP-UP (CONTINUED)

Glossary

complacency What occurs when you believe you are so good at your job that you stop thinking about how to do it properly.

sensorimotor cues Sights, sounds, and smells that create an awareness of environmental conditions; this awareness may prompt a behavioral response.

References

1. Maguire BJ, Hunting KL, Smith GS, Levick NR. Occupational fatalities in emergency medical services: a hidden crisis. *Ann Emer Med.* 2002;40:625–632.

2. Maguire BJ, Smith S. Injuries and fatalities among emergency medical technicians in the United States. *Prehosp Disaster Med.* 2013;28(4):376–382.

Suggested Readings

1. De Castro AB. Handle with care: The American Nurses Association campaign to address work-related musculoskeletal disorders. *Online Journal of Issues in Nursing.* 2004;9(3):3.

CHAPTER 2

Crew Resource Management

© Barbol/Shutterstock

CHAPTER OBJECTIVES

After reading this chapter, the participant will be able to:

- Describe the origins of crew resource management (CRM)

- Describe the goals of crew resource management

- Describe the role of teamwork within crew resource management

- Describe the core traits of a leader within crew resource management

- Explain the strategies to maintain situational awareness

- Identify the common factors that lead to the loss of situational awareness

- Describe the key elements of open communication within crew resource management

- Explain what leads to human error and how to reduce errors

© Barbol/Shutterstock

SCENARIO

You're working the night shift as a field training officer, and your partner is "a newbie." Your unit is dispatched to a patient in respiratory distress. On your arrival at a single-family home, you are directed upstairs where, in the back bedroom, you find a 44-year-old male in severe respiratory distress. The patient is morbidly obese, at over 500 pounds. He is sweating heavily, unable to speak in full sentences, and a quick assessment of his lung sounds shows bilateral crackles.

While you and your partner are having a quick discussion on the best course of treatment and how you're going to move the patient safely to the ambulance, the patient goes into respiratory arrest. You realize there are a dozen things that need to be done immediately, including managing the patient's airway, figuring out how to get him out to the ambulance safely, and dealing with his upset family.

Your partner contacts the dispatcher and requests additional resources. Shortly, a fire engine, two police cars, and another ambulance show up to assist you. An EMS supervisor is en route as well. The fire captain tells you that they're going to bring in a rescue company to move the patient. A member of the ambulance crew argues that the patient should be moved immediately. His partner begins arguing with the patient's mother about which hospital the patient will be transferred to, while the police officers are trying to usher the rest of the family out of the bedroom.

1. What are your primary nonclinical priorities?
2. What is one of the best tools you have at your disposal to manage the scene?
3. How do you deal with conflicting opinions on the best course of treatment?

Introduction

Emergency medical services (EMS) practitioners all need to speak up when it comes to safety because poor communication, weak teamwork, and bravado are the top causes of injuries and line-of-duty deaths.[1] So the question is, why don't we, as EMS practitioners, speak up when we see something out of place or have an alternative solution based on previous experiences? All too often, EMS has created an environment where the communication path travels in one direction, from the senior authority on down to the trainee. In addition, EMS practitioners may not speak up because of a fear of being wrong, reprisal, and embarrassment. By implementing crew resource management, EMS agencies can ensure that communication paths remain open and that all EMS practitioners at every level of position and experience feel empowered to communicate. The collective goal is safety and for all EMS practitioners to be engaged and responsible for the safety of their partners, their crew, and their patients.

Crew Resource Management

Crew resource management (CRM) is a tool originally instituted by the airline industry in the 1980s to optimize performance and outcomes by reducing the effect of human error through the use of all available resources. After an airline crash in 1978 in Portland, Oregon, which was the result of

poor collective situational awareness, failures in team communication, and misunderstandings about the fuel system, the airline industry developed CRM training for their airline crews FIGURE 2-1 . The goal of CRM training is to enable high-performance teams, such as airline or ambulance crews, to achieve and maintain collective situational awareness. Situational awareness is the state of being aware of what is happening in order to understand how information, events, and a person's actions will affect his or her goals and objectives, both now and in the near future.

CRM has been adopted by many high-reliability organizations (HROs) and other industries, including EMS and fire, in an effort to reduce injuries and accidents and improve patient care. HROs are organizations that operate in high-risk environments, such as those associated with law enforcement, fire and EMS, power and utilities, chemical factories, and air traffic control. A common trait among HROs is that their margin for error is minuscule, and the fallout from an adverse event could be disastrous. Critical HRO components include mindfulness, an inclination toward inquiry and doubt as a means of evaluating and updating standard procedures, attention to the complexities of an emergency incident, commitment to resilience, and a willingness to defer to expertise.

CRM Components

When groups of competent, trained individuals get together to solve problems, they typically define the issue and then deploy a combination of "humanware," software, and hardware to solve the problem. In this context, software implementation can be rewriting training manuals or procedures or developing

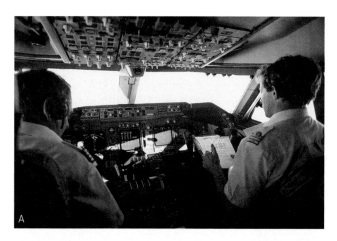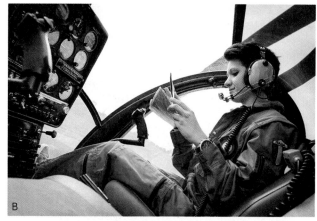

Figure 2-1 **A.** CRM was developed by the airline industry to improve collective situational awareness and communication among the airplane's crew. **B.** CRM is applied throughout EMS, including critical care transport.

(A) © Hauke Dressler/LOOK-foto/Getty; (B) © pio3/Shutterstock

IN THE FIELD

Another concept developed by the airline industry is the "sterile cockpit." In the sterile cockpit, during key points in the flight, such as take-off and landing, the sole focus of the pilots' attention should be on the task at hand. To apply this to EMS, when the emergency vehicle operator is driving, his or her focus should be purely on driving the vehicle. The emergency vehicle operator should not be distracted by navigating or radio chatter.

checklists and policies. **Hardware** solutions can take the form of the use of computers, vehicles, tools, medications, or protective equipment. The **humanware** component consists of those people who are part of a team and have been directed to solve a particular problem—for example, a patient in respiratory arrest. EMS agencies with open communication and that embrace respectful and informed feedback as a method for encouraging collective situational awareness develop skills for their humanware to solve complex problems effectively within dynamic environments—for example, an ambulance crew working together to assess and care for a patient in cardiac arrest in the crowded chaos of a county fair. Essentially, EMS agencies that practice CRM build up the communication skills of their EMS practitioners and ingrain these skills into daily practice.

Simply embracing an open communication environment and encouraging collaboration does not address all the differences in individual behavior and communication styles. An experienced and seasoned EMS practitioner who is part of a problem-solving team understands that he or she will make little progress if the human team members are unable to communicate effectively.

Incident Command System

The **incident command system (ICS)** is used during both emergency incidents as well as preplanned events to help identify incident needs and priorities. By identifying roles and responsibilities, outlining clear lines of communication, limiting the span of control, and providing methods for expanding the incident, a well-developed incident command system allows leaders and managers to deploy resources in a structured and objective manner **FIGURE 2-2**. However, implementing ICS is not a guarantee that the incident will be resolved flawlessly.

What CRM can provide to ICS is behavioral expectations for the humanware involved in the incident. Because CRM uses a specific model of seeking input, acknowledging communication, respectfully providing differing opinions, resolving conflict, and monitoring a decision, CRM can highlight the areas where team communication breaks down. In addition, by analyzing the team's performance postincident and looking for the moments when team communications became ineffective, an EMS agency can design specific strategies for improvement.

IN THE FIELD

The success of CRM depends on its acceptance by the entire EMS agency. To ensure that every EMS practitioner starts and stays on the same page, laying a solid foundation in the tools of CRM is necessary. This foundation includes training personnel in the techniques of open and respectful communication, developing a comprehensive approach to identifying and tracking errors and mistakes, educating and training personnel in conflict management, and instituting regular and recurring critiques so that members can learn from each other.

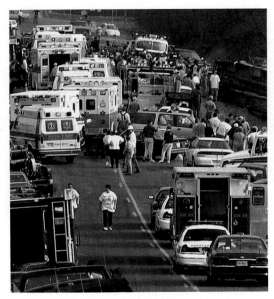

Figure 2-2 The incident command system (ICS) allows leaders and managers to deploy resources in a structured and objective manner.

© David Crigger, Bristol Herald Courier/AP Images

IN THE FIELD

ICS utilizes some of the principles of CRM. As with the incident commander in ICS, in CRM, there is only one leader, and that team leader retains the ultimate decision-making authority. Just as an incident commander listens to the information relayed by branch directors, the CRM leader processes inputs from the rest of the team to render more efficient and correct decisions. Leaders versed in CRM recognize their limits and encourage their subordinates to participate in the decision-making process. This results in a greater understanding of the goals and objectives by everyone involved and keeps the team mission oriented.

IN THE FIELD

When an EMS agency needs to determine who should be driving the ambulances, the decision should not be made in a vacuum. Safety managers may review existing policies (software), use driver simulation systems (hardware), and review driver performance under direct observation (humanware) **FIGURE 2-3**. They may also look at support agencies for recommendations on how to evaluate a safe driver—for example, an insurance carrier.

Number of Violations (Last Five Years)	Number of Accidents (Last Five Years)			
	0	**1**	**2**	**3 (or more)**
No Minor Violations	Clear	OK to Drive	Borderline	Cannot Drive
1 Minor Violation*	OK to Drive	OK to Drive	Borderline	Cannot Drive
2 Minor Violations	OK to Drive	Borderline	Cannot Drive	Cannot Drive
3 Minor Violations	Borderline	Cannot Drive	Cannot Drive	Cannot Drive
4 or More Minor Violations	Cannot Drive	Cannot Drive	Cannot Drive	Cannot Drive
Any Major Violation**	Cannot Drive	Cannot Drive	Cannot Drive	Cannot Drive

*Note: Minor violations can be defined as any moving violation except: motor vehicle equipment, load, or size requirements; improper or failure to display license plates; failure to sign or display registration; failure to have driver's license in possession; or a minor violation in which the driver has been charged with an accident

**Note: Major violations can be defined as: driving under the influence; driving while impaired; failure to stop or report an accident; reckless driving or a speeding contest; homicide, manslaughter, or arrest arising out of the use of a vehicle; making a false accident report; driving with a suspended or revoked license; attempting to elude a police officer

Figure 2-3 An example of a decision matrix (Courtesy of MONOC Mobile Health Services).

Teamwork

Within high-performance teams, regular use of CRM to gain a shared understanding continually improves performance FIGURE 2-4 . Specifically, when teams practice communication techniques that are designed to share understanding, members have opportunities to build team discipline, broaden the knowledge base of individual team members, and remove boundaries to learning. Additionally, CRM can establish trust and respect within teams, reduce the chance for error caused by distraction, and encourage collective situational awareness.

Because CRM is an interactive process, the roles of each team member must be clearly communicated. It is also vital to know who is leading the team. In CRM, although every team member's voice is important, and each person's role is vital to the team's success, there is one leader.

Team members should understand each other's roles and responsibilities. By "cross-pollinating," team members learn whom to turn to when specific problems arise, reducing the risk of one team member reaching the point of task overload. By sharing what their roles are with each other, team members become more likely to speak out if someone becomes overwhelmed by tasks or if they believe a fellow team member may have missed a cue that is important to his or her individual task and the team's collective success.

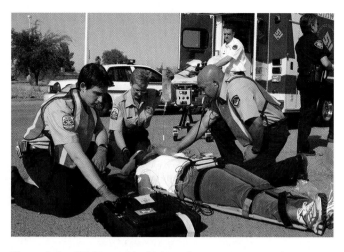

Figure 2-4 CRM is used by high-performance teams, such as EMS, to reduce injuries and accidents through teamwork and open communication.

© Jones & Bartlett Learning. Courtesy of MIEMSS.

IN THE FIELD

A team is composed of everyone who is working as a group to solve the problem at hand. It can be a small team—for example, two paramedics on an ambulance, four fire fighters on an engine, or two police officers in a police car—or it can be all eight emergency responders working together. Teams can involve multiple agencies from multiple jurisdictions.

Conflict and Respect

Good teams develop a level of trust that goes beyond technical expertise. They actually come to understand the importance of collectively solving problems, and they value the diversity of opinions within the team. Diverse opinions, in any team, lead to some level of conflict. In this context, conflict is not bad. Instead, the success or failure of a team often depends on how the team manages conflict and whether team members are able to benefit from conflict by using it to outline strategic differences.

The trust developed within a team using CRM is based predominantly on the core value of respect. Every team member, when confronting an idea, action, order, or behavior, must exhibit respect for his or her fellow members regardless of rank, position within the team, or level of expertise.

Leaders

Leaders can become leaders based on a legal statute or position of authority (e.g., EMS chief), or an EMS practitioner can assume a leadership role based on ability. The core behaviors of an effective leader are:

- Envisioning goals and setting clear objectives
- Delegating authority
- Taking responsibility
- Gaining commitment and motivating the team
- Maintaining situational awareness
- Understanding individual and team limitations
- Possessing the ability to adjust to the situation
- Valuing team diversity
- Having the ability to listen aggressively and with curiosity
- Setting clear expectations

IN THE FIELD

Knowing the limits or the strengths and weaknesses of the team and its members will allow leaders to capitalize on the team members' strengths and minimize the effects of any weakness. Lifting and moving is one example. If one team member has greater upper body strength than another, that will impact the positions that each member takes during a lift.

Most teams are created for a specific purpose—to get something done. The team leader typically needs to consider the number and types of objectives, their clarity, and their priority, with input from team members. Because there are often competing objectives and multiple methods for achieving them, effective leaders communicate what they perceive to be the priorities and then ask for input. They set a direction for the team. This ability requires the following skills:

1. Leaders must be able to get the team's attention and hold it while distractions occur.

    Gaining and holding the team's attention can be done using hierarchy (the leader's authority position), but a leader usually has more success by employing subtle people skills. For example, some leaders have been very successful in getting and holding the team's attention by using steady eye contact and a quiet, calm tone of voice that requires the team members to listen actively. This method also can help reduce the tension level.

IN THE FIELD

Not everyone can be a leader; some people have to be followers, and this should not be taken as a negative sentiment. All good leaders have high-performance followers. The followers enable the leader to focus on the big picture. Followers also have a role to be prepared, engaged, and focused members of the crew. Just as leaders have responsibilities, so do followers, including:

- Ensuring safety
- Accepting and following directions
- Being prepared physically and mentally
- Recognizing limitations of self and others
- Focusing on teamwork
- Having a positive attitude
- Being flexible

Success depends on the entire team, not just the leader. After all, it is the followers who will implement the leader's plans and act as additional eyes and ears.

Look at a typical emergency services organizational structure. There is a chief, and this individual sets the direction for the agency and sets the tone on the importance of safety in the field, with clear preventive policies and procedures. It is the responsibility of the "followers" or the deputy chiefs to implement the chief's directions via policies and protocols. The field staff, who are also followers, actually ensure that preventive policies and procedures are implemented on a shift-by-shift basis. Without followers, preventive policies and procedures will not succeed.

Remember, a leader without people following is just a person out taking a walk.

2. Leaders must be able to gain situational awareness, identify goals, and set specific and achievable objectives.

    Strong leaders understand that goals can be identified only after they have a sense of what is happening and what needs to be done. Situational awareness in a team environment requires activating a feedback loop: asking for input, requesting updates, and checking in with each individual. An important point to remember is that leaders should expect to receive unpleasant information if they openly ask for input. The news they receive may not be what they anticipate, yet it is critical that leaders maintain a sense of active curiosity, particularly if they perceive something differently from how a reporting team member perceives it.

3. Leaders must have the ability to ensure that all team members understand the team's stated goals and objectives.

    Misunderstandings are common in team communication. Good leaders desire a shared understanding among team members in which goals and objectives have a common definition. Leaders can achieve shared understanding by asking team members to restate the specific goal or objective. Questions such as "What do you think we need to do now?" help provide clarification, particularly if the goal includes multiple steps or requires the involvement of other teams for a successful outcome.

Situational Awareness

Situational awareness has three primary components: an awareness of the surroundings and how individuals are supposed to interact with the surroundings; the reality of the situation; and individual perceptions of the situation. Situational awareness is an internal active evaluation process that goes on constantly, much like size-up. EMS practitioners must update their situational awareness constantly by observing their surroundings, evaluating their options, and communicating with those around them.

The dynamic, fluid emergencies that EMS practitioners respond to require that they maintain the absolute highest state of alertness and attention at all times **FIGURE 2-5**. Because EMS practitioners are human, loss of situational awareness does occur. This loss of situational awareness is common when they perform routine tasks in familiar surroundings. As EMS practitioners gain experience, they often pay less attention to the mundane details of everyday operations. But these details can become important as a situation becomes complex.

Maintaining situational awareness is a skill that can be taught. Essentially, the following behaviors help teams maintain situational awareness:

- Ask yourself, "What can go wrong?" This should be a challenging question. What poses the biggest risk? What is the smallest risk? What would happen if either of those things occurred? How would you work with your team to regain control of the situation?

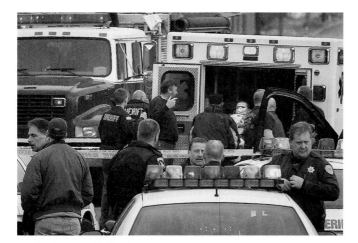

Figure 2-5 The chaotic and complex emergencies that EMS practitioners respond to require that they maintain the absolute highest state of alertness and attention at all times.

© Jason Hunt/The Coeur d'Alene Press/AP Photo

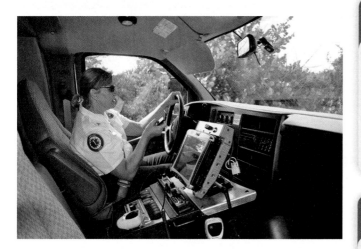

Figure 2-6 Emergency vehicle operators should be completely focused on driving, not distractions such as cell phones.

Courtesy of Sunstar Paramedics.

- Reducing the opportunity for unnecessary distraction. On the way to the call, cell phones should be off, and you should be focusing on the information that dispatch has shared **FIGURE 2-6**.
- Regularly stating the primary mission of the team. Once distracted, a team can head off in a direction that results in a critical loss of situational awareness. This is directly tied to the concept of "Who's flying the plane?" Pilots know that regardless of the number of distractions, their primary mission is still to fly the plane. In a medical context, this can be stated as: "Let's bag the patient. A, B, C, let's not forget the basics."

The following are several of the more common factors that lead to distraction or loss of situational awareness.

- **Ambiguous statements or situations.** Team members who make ambiguous statements are usually trying to make sense of their surroundings or the situation. They often see something that doesn't fit, and their statements are designed to express concern without overtly stating that they don't know what's going on. Pay attention to random, ambiguous statements and "close the loop" by asking for clarification. "What specifically is your concern? What do you see that is bothering you?" These types of questions help provide clarity and understanding. Ambiguous statements can also include inconsistent terminology, which is why it is vital to use plain text instead of slang when speaking. Ambiguity in situations must also be brought out and clearly stated. For example, if it isn't clear who is responsible for picking up the gear at the end of a call, ask, "Would you like me to pack up?" If a statement or situation appears ambiguous, work to provide clarity.

IN THE FIELD

Maintaining situational awareness is a continuous process as the surrounding environment changes. We need to be cognizant of the clues that tell us change is about to happen—a large crowd forming around us as we treat the patient or the changes in the rhythm on the EKG monitor.

IN THE FIELD

EMS agencies should develop concise procedures for unusual occurrences **TABLE 2-1**. Having a detailed procedure written ahead of time and staff trained on these procedures reduces the likelihood of deviation and the resultant negative consequences.

Table 2-1 Special Situations Requiring SOPs	
Helicopter responses	WMD
Large-scale incidents	Large venues
Special populations	Natural disasters
IED responses	Hazardous materials
SWAT requests	Fires

■ **Implementing an improper procedure or not following a good one.** When is it appropriate to deviate from procedures? Ideally, procedures are designed to keep EMS practitioners and their patients safe. Policies and procedures spell out what EMS practitioners are expected to do in certain situations, and in some cases, they only provide a framework to achieve a goal or objective. Vigilance is needed to combat the urge to take shortcuts or do it "my way." Such an attitude not only puts EMS practitioners and the patients at risk for harm but also puts the EMS agency and EMS practitioners at risk of litigation. Remember, policies cannot address all the subtle differences that occur in emergency situations. Experienced EMS practitioners must determine the best method for implementing procedures that are designed to help them achieve a good outcome.

■ **Failure to deal with distraction.** Dealing with distraction is an art form developed over time. EMS practitioners need to regularly ask about the removal of distracting elements. Will removing certain elements reduce their overall situational awareness or contribute to their ability to concentrate on the most important tasks and objectives? For example, while driving, is the emergency vehicle operator distracted by the radio, mobile data terminal, cell phone, GPS system, pager, conversation with a partner, or his or her emotions? A simple action such as cutting down on nonessential conversation removes distraction and allows all team members to be aware of things in their environment that could compromise safety.

■ **Fixation on a single objective.** Fixation is common when there are multiple distractions. One method humans use to improve performance is to consciously block out things that are not directly tied to our primary objective. In EMS, it takes the form of EMS practitioners paying so much attention to one procedure that they ignore other important cues—for example, treating the bleeding from a gunshot wound but not considering who shot the patient and where they are now.

■ **Complacency.** Few people come to work wanting to be labeled as complacent. Yet, in accident reports, complacency is often listed as a cause. Complacency itself is not an accident cause; it is an effect. Complacency is the effect of a sense of comfort with certain routine procedures or practices. These procedures or practices are done so often and within the same environment that EMS practitioners often lose sight of their importance. This is especially evident with safety practices that are allowed to go unchecked, such as seat belt use, appropriate glove use, and use of personal protective equipment.

■ **Failure to resolve or properly manage conflicts or conflicting conditions.** EMS practitioners need

IN THE FIELD

One of the elements the airline industry developed to combat complacency is the checklist. A pilot may have 10,000 hours in the cockpit with zero adverse events, but before every take-off and every landing, he or she reviews the proper procedures using a checklist that details the steps that must be completed to ensure a successful take-off, flight, and landing. This is something that EMS practitioners should adopt when performing high-risk or complicated procedures such as rapid sequence intubation.

IN THE FIELD

In January 2006, David Rosenbaum suffered a critical head injury during a mugging in Washington, D.C. Fire fighters and EMTs responded and found him unconscious on the sidewalk. He was quickly assessed and incorrectly assumed to be intoxicated and without associated injury. This complacent assessment and failure to follow protocol resulted in a significant delay in Mr. Rosenbaum's transport and treatment. Mr. Rosenbaum, a prominent *New York Times* reporter, later died of his injuries. The national media took interest in the case because it seemed to highlight the issue of complacency in EMS.

to pay close attention to managing conflict. In many cases, the conflict is communications based. Conflict is a normal, helpful part of collective problem solving if it is managed correctly. This means ensuring people are heard, repeating the message back to ensure it was heard correctly, and maintaining respect among team members. If there are conflicting conditions, team members must call attention to the conflicts so that shared understanding of the priorities and goals can develop.

■ **Task overload.** It is often said that if something needs to be done, give the job to a busy person. But this is a dangerous tactic in EMS. The workload needs to be balanced between team members whenever possible. For example, an emergency vehicle operator should be focused on the road, not talking to dispatch or navigating. Task overload can also refer to information overload. A self-protective mechanism kicks in, and the mind starts shutting down; if the mind is no longer paying attention, details get overlooked. Sometimes a response to overload is a noncaring attitude similar to burnout. When this occurs, it is time to slow down the momentum ever so slightly and prioritize. "Okay, what needs to be done next?"

- **"No one is flying the plane."** It is important to clarify what CRM is not designed for. CRM is not team decision making. Every team needs a leader, and the leader is tasked with carefully listening to input, evaluating the options, leading any discussion if there is conflict, and ultimately making the decision regarding which course of action is appropriate. The team provides open, honest, respectful input, but the leader decides on the course of action.

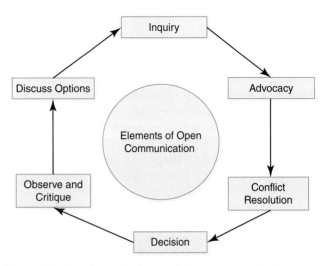

Figure 2-7 The elements of successful open communication are inquiry, advocacy, conflict resolution, decision, observe and critique, and discuss options.

© Jones & Bartlett Learning.

IN THE FIELD

Errors can occur when someone is task overloaded, so constraints must be put in place to prevent this from happening. A simple strategy is to divide the workload into manageable parts. This promotes teamwork, provides increased margin of safety, and encourages strategies for handling overload. For example, during the response phase of a call, let the driver be responsible for driving. Have the partner work the radios and program the mapping system. Whenever possible, make sure you have the correct resources and necessary personnel.

IN THE FIELD

One of the areas that CRM attempts to correct is communication errors. Have you ever been dispatched to "123 Main"? Or to "the basketball court"? When you attempted to clarify the address with dispatch, did you get an unhelpful response? CRM attempts to look at all the factors involved in communication issues and solve the problem, as opposed to punishing or assigning blame.

Open Communications

The typical CRM model contains several key elements, all of which are integral to gaining a shared understanding in a culture of learning and mutual respect. These elements are inquiry, advocacy, conflict resolution, decision, observe and critique, and discuss options FIGURE 2-7 . In a typical incident, these elements are used in a seamless communication process. Once the steps have been practiced, team members often do not consciously walk through each one; instead, they use the process automatically, as part of the fabric of an open communication model that allows a shared understanding among team members.

Inquiry

The first step in the CRM circle of successful communication is inquiry. Good practices during the inquiry phase include aggressive listening skills, allowing an environment in which respectful commentary is accepted, and carefully intervening to ensure that the question is heard correctly.

An inquiry typically comes across in one of the following forms:

- A statement by a team member or the team leader: "This is our objective, to lift this patient up this staircase, and here is how we are going to do it."
- An order from a superior: "Give 50 mg of Benadryl IM"
- An action: A team member, leader or otherwise, performs an action that draws the attention of other team members.

All team members should remember that a statement is declarative. If a statement is made by a superior or someone with more experience or expertise than the team member on the receiving end of the spoken message, the receiver often misunderstands the statement as an order or a demand. However, it is important for team members to understand that statements are simply declarations of fact or observation and that they can still be questioned.

Coherence

One of the most common errors made at the inquiry stage results from miscommunication associated with coherence. **Coherence** is associated with how well the receiver understands the message. Coherence is possible when the truth of a situation aligns with the words spoken by the sender. In some cases, the sender means one thing and the receiver hears another because the sender may be using terminology that is unfamiliar to the receiver or that has one meaning to the sender and another to the receiver.

Coherence can also be a problem when different agencies use different signals, procedures, or terms. Sometimes this can even occur within the same organization. For instance, an EMS practitioner might be asked to "give 10 of Benadryl." Did the sender mean 10 milligrams or 10 milliliters? In most cases, the difference in meaning is significant and needs to be clarified.

The best way to deal with terminology coherence issues is for team members to practice repeating back what they think they heard or what they understand to be correct, not exactly what the person said. "I understand you want 10 milliliters of Benadryl, or 50 milligrams. Is that correct?" For procedural differences, it is best in advance of any incident to collaborate with various agencies to standardize regional practices and procedures, particularly those related to safety.

Advocacy

In many typical CRM structures, the second step in the communication loop is labeled advocacy. However, advocacy does little to actually describe the process that occurs when a team member feels a disconnect with something he or she has heard or seen in the inquiry phase. Questioning authority is a daunting task. During this step, it is crucial for team members to understand that there are two methods for approving of an action or statement they see or hear, and only one method for providing a **challenge**. The two methods of providing approval for the actions or statements of others are to verbally state understanding and agreement and to voice no objection at all.

The second method of indicating approval, saying nothing, is all too common—and too commonly misused, as becomes apparent during postincident analyses. During critiques, team members might wonder how much understanding was truly shared at the incident. For example, a team member will state that he or she had a concern, or "knew" something was going to happen, but the person typically had a reason for not speaking up. Leaders are often astonished when they hear this. Why didn't the person voice an opinion? Leaders assume that everyone approves after they have asked for input and no one voices an objection.

PACE

One method that can help all EMS practitioners practice advocacy was first developed for airline crews so they could effectively challenge seasoned captains. The acronym PACE describes a series of actions that team members can take to make better sense of what they see and hear **FIGURE 2-8** :

- **Probe** for better understanding (the **sense-making** phase).
- **Alert** the leader to any concerns or abnormalities.
- **Challenge** the suitability of a current action or strategy if the probe and alert do not appear to be changing the course of action.
- **Emergency intervention** if there is critical danger and the team continues on a course that will cause harm.

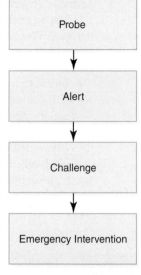

Figure 2-8 The acronym PACE describes a series of actions that team members can take to make better sense of what they see and hear.

© Jones & Bartlett Learning.

Conflict Resolution

Few people truly enjoy conflict, yet it is a necessary part of team dynamics and a by-product of bringing together any group of high-performance individuals with experience and strong opinions. Add the components of personal danger, time pressure, and a high-stakes outcome, and it is a recipe for poor performance. However, it is not the absence of conflict that makes a good team but the manner in which team members handle it. The key to conflict resolution revolves around the saying "what is right, not who is right." **Conflict resolution** is a range of processes aimed at alleviating or eliminating sources of conflict; these generally include negotiation, mediation, and diplomacy. It is important to remember that CRM is not team decision making. Most teams using CRM principles are not formed on democratic principles but instead have a hierarchy related to training, position, and experience. It is critically important for team members to understand how they should handle conflict when it inevitably occurs.

A cardinal rule in conflict resolution—and one of the most difficult to employ—is for team members to stay focused on the mission or the issue at hand. Therefore, all participants must continually remind themselves to devote all attention to the current source of conflict. Conflict resolution is not the place to address past disputes. Biases need to be put aside. The primary goal is for everyone involved to concentrate all efforts on resolution.

IN THE FIELD

Remember to keep your speech clear, concise, informative, and direct.

When managing conflict at this stage in the CRM communication loop, it is helpful to understand that complete resolution of the conflict is not likely to occur until after the situation is entirely concluded, and more time can be spent discussing options. It is important to remember that this loop often takes only seconds to complete in real-time situations. In the midst of any incident, the most anyone can hope for is to achieve an understanding of what the concerns are and why they exist. Sometimes the best that team leaders and decision makers can do, particularly if they are not planning on changing the strategy even after hearing the concern, is to communicate clearly to the individual expressing the concern that they understand what he or she is saying, recognize the potential impact, and value the input.

Decision

As indicated, the primary reason to employ CRM principles is to provide a collective situational awareness to the team. There must be an identified leader on every team who can make decisions. Teams without leaders tend to wander among options, with no one person assuming responsibility for the team's actions or the outcome.

One of the duties of a good leader is to take responsibility for team performance. Good leaders are decisive, yet they are also empathetic and careful listeners. A decision should be made when team members get behind the group's efforts, even if one of them does not necessarily agree with the chosen course.

During the next phase of observe and critique, team members need to provide input because the entire team witnesses events unfold after a decision is made. Additionally, leaders must keep in mind that during critical communication events, many decisions are made, and the constant flow of communication is critical. If a leader and the team have reevaluated their strategy and decided to employ a new one, it is imperative that the entire team be aware of this, along with anyone else who may be affected. Decision making carries with it a great responsibility.

Observe and Critique

After the decision has been made to move forward with a particular strategy, it is important for all team members to carefully observe the process and evaluate progress against the initially stated mission goals. If something appears unsafe, if things aren't going according to plan, or if the individuals or equipment chosen for the task don't appear appropriate, a good team engages in critique conversation in which they evaluate the situation on the fly. This should be constructive conversation and should include specifics: What isn't working as expected? Why might the problem exist? What can be done to modify the plan? These brief yet important communications lead to discussing options.

Observation leads to critique, and critique should be an open process because it brings out comments, statements, and questions that lead the team to discuss options, guiding back to the inquiry phase. This is where good leaders shine: They encourage input, particularly when things start to get quiet. If team members are not commenting on their observations, they aren't collectively sharing their understanding of what they see.

Discuss Options

As the team members critique their work and its results, they may decide that other options are necessary. In critical situations that develop over a period of time, this duty is often relegated to a planning section. Within the small team environment and during rapidly developing situations, options are often presented as questions that are posed to the group. Options are a necessary part of emergency operations in any dynamic environment. EMS practitioners must recognize that even though a team has determined a course of action, team members must always evaluate other options. In this context, many team leaders start ordering resources and planning logistically to implement one of several alternatives.

Discussing options moves the team back into the beginning phase of the CRM loop: They had a plan, they made a decision on what to do, they evaluated their evolving circumstances, and they proposed options and outlined risk. The new option returns to the beginning of the process and is considered an inquiry ("What do you think of Plan B?"), and team members can openly agree with the idea or probe further to develop any concerns.

IN THE FIELD

Don't assume that communication is based only on your words. Your body language and nonverbal cues are also important. Not making eye contact or having a defensive posture can be interpreted as "This person is not being honest with me."

IN THE FIELD

When you are communicating, keep these questions in mind:

- Did you hear what was said?
- Did you repeat back what was said?
- Are there language barriers?
- Is everyone using the same terminology?
- Are you asking the right questions?
- Are you being passive or aggressive?
- Are you afraid to speak up to ask clarifying questions?

Decision Making

Emergency scenes are event-driven scenarios. This means that every situation unfolds in a manner that is relatively unpredictable and that the tempo of events is not entirely under the control of the EMS practitioners. In addition, each person viewing the exact same scene will have a slightly different perspective based in part on that person's area of expertise, level of experience, quality of training, ability to recall applicable procedures, and personal context. Members of any group on an emergency scene do, however, share two significant realities: No one knows exactly how the situation will unfold, and no one knows the outcome.

High-performance teams work best when they have a collective understanding of the situation they face. Effective CRM ensures that every member of the team has an appreciation of the following key points:

- The exact nature of the problem, its cause, and any confounding or complicating factors
- The skills, strengths, weaknesses, and experience of their fellow team members
- An understanding of what is likely to happen based on taking no action
- An understanding of what is likely to happen if the team chooses a specific action
- A shared knowledge of the desired outcome
- A shared strategy, with an understanding of what needs to be accomplished, by whom, and when
- The knowledge that any member of the team, regardless of training, position, or experience, can respectfully question the strategy and/or provide additional cues that will help the team gain a better understanding of the situation as it unfolds

Only when the team truly knows how to use CRM can it maximize the potential for a successful outcome. Gaining the ability to develop and cultivate a shared vision among team members is a skill that requires practice and knowledge of how

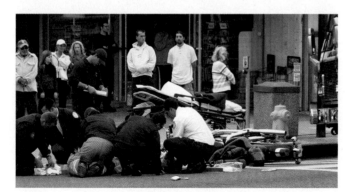

Figure 2-9 Unlike in situations where people have the benefit of time, emergency work is extremely dynamic and fast paced.
© Michael Ledray/ShutterStock, Inc.

the human mind works while under pressure to make a decision. Unlike in situations in which people have the benefit of time and know that an outcome will be the same every time they apply a set of rules and procedures, emergency work is extremely dynamic FIGURE 2-9 . EMS practitioners cannot know every factor influencing the emergency situation before they must make a decision, and they must be able to adjust and adapt as the situation unfolds. Team members should know when and how to slightly slow the decision process to gain a better perspective.

Reducing Human Error

Incident investigation finds that errors are not random in EMS. People cause accidents by making errors. Errors arise from poor communication, poor teamwork, and not paying attention. By mitigating errors, EMS practitioners can reduce deaths and injuries. One of the basic goals of CRM is to reduce errors because errors are costly to both an EMS agency and EMS practitioners. In the event of a collision, the EMS agency may lose the use of the vehicle or incur the cost of repairs, lawsuits, and worker compensation claims. If an ambulance crew member is injured, he or she may suffer lost wages or a permanent disability.

Errors Are Not Random

Errors are predictable, and situations that are predictable are preventable. In the 1930s, H. W. Heinrich, an industrial safety pioneer, reported on a study of accidents that he classified according to severity. Heinrich's report showed that for each serious-injury incident, we could expect to see that the same type of error caused about 29 minor injuries and 300 near-miss or property-damage-only incidents. This is commonly referred to as Heinrich's Law.[2]

When applying the ratios suggested by Heinrich, it has been recommended that the focus of safety programs be on preventing less serious events as an indirect means to prevent a single serious event. Is it always true that serious injuries are caused by the same factors that cause less serious incidents? Many experts believe that this is the case. This is the reasoning behind near-miss reporting. If the factors that led to a near miss can be identified, then policies can be put in place to ensure that those factors do not occur again. Ignoring the lessons of a near miss will eventually lead to a serious-injury incident.

Risk Assessment

Through a risk assessment, EMS practitioners can identify specific work processes and perform a simple evaluation of the associated risk. To conduct a risk assessment, EMS practitioners need to first identify what hazards exist in the workplace. For example, driving with lights and sirens, handling contaminated sharps, and loading and unloading patients are all hazardous tasks that EMS practitioners perform on a daily basis. Next, EMS practitioners look at each hazard and determine the potential

NAEMT, in collaboration with the Center for Leadership, Innovation, and Research in EMS, developed an anonymous system for EMS practitioners to report near-miss, line-of-duty death, and patient safety incidents by answering a series of questions in an online format. This reporting system is called the EMS Voluntary Event Notification Tool (EVENT) and is available at their website.

The purpose of the system is to collect and aggregate data that are then analyzed and used in the development of EMS policies and procedures, and for use in training, educating, and preventing similar events from occurring in the future. No individual responses are shared or transmitted to other parties. The aggregated data collected are provided to state EMS offices and the appropriate federal agencies with jurisdiction over EMS on a quarterly and annual basis.

Heinrich promoted the concept of focusing on controlling hazards in the workplace in addition to changing worker behaviors. He also found that accidents share certain commonalities—policy violation, lack of training, and unclear directions. If these issues can be addressed at the earliest and most basic level, then future events can be prevented.

risks associated with it. For example, with contaminated sharps, EMS practitioners would examine a pathway in which staff were harmed, such as being stuck with a dirty needle. EMS practitioners also need to look at the incidents in which staff are stuck with a clean needle. Next, examine how the needle sticks occurred: Was it during the IV attempt or transference of the needle to the sharps container? Was the ambulance crew provided with the proper education on how to use the device and how to safely dispose of it? Did staff violate the safeguards of the device or violate a policy? Was the device defective? As the cause is investigated, issues can be identified and corrected by revising training, updating policies, or changing the type of needle used.

A constant review by managers of incident reports, lawsuits, customer complaints, worker compensation reports, biomedical information, fleet reports, and clinical counseling files may indicate patterns or trends that can be used to identify potential fail points. Once issues are identified, they can be corrected by

changing a process, piece of equipment, or procedure. The corrective focus should be on those behaviors that can be labeled a high risk. Simply ask: How likely is it to happen, and how bad will it be if it does happen?

Personal Strategies

There are personal strategies for error reduction. First, ensure a high level of proficiency in your knowledge and skills. Understand your policies and procedures. Have open communications and ensure that everyone on the team knows that he or she can call a safety time-out if things are not clear. For example, if a lifting and moving plan isn't clear, you should stop before "Ready, one, two, three" is called to clarify what your role is.

Minimize distractions in order to allow yourself to focus on the task at hand and use the concepts within CRM to maintain situational awareness. Recognize that technology has its limitations, and unless the equipment is properly maintained, it will not function correctly. Last, accept that most errors are due to humans, which is why it is critical to be a high-functioning member of a high-functioning team.

Postincident Analysis (PIA)

Postincident analysis (PIA) is an activity that takes place after the incident to review the team's performance and the validity of current policies and focuses on identifying the lessons learned FIGURE 2-10 . As discussed previously, the factors that lead to a near miss or minor accident can lead to a serious injury or death during another incident. The PIA is an opportunity to identify issues that may be occurring on a daily basis to prevent minor or major errors from occurring.

For example, a critical care ambulance performs an interfacility transport with a patient destined for a cardiac catheterization lab. On removing the patient from the ambulance,

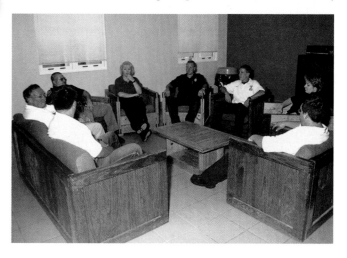

Figure 2-10 The PIA is an opportunity to identify issues that may be occurring on a daily basis in order to prevent minor or major errors from occurring.

the stretcher collapses to the ground. The patient states that he is not injured when questioned by the EMS practitioners. The patient is then brought to the catheterization lab for his scheduled procedure. Later that afternoon, the patient's family notifies the EMS agency of the incident. Several weeks later, a notice of claim is received by the EMS agency because the patient intends to sue. Additionally, the family lodges a complaint with the Department of Health, which in turn conducts its own investigation.

A PIA reveals that there was a last-minute crew change as the ambulance went into service. The fleet of critical care ambulances used a different model of stretcher than the Basic Life Support (BLS) division did, and the EMS practitioner was not familiar with the loading and unloading process with the stretcher. After the accident, the crew followed the EMS agency's policy and generated an incident report but did not notify the supervisor of this event. In addition, the crew members did not obtain a refusal of medical attention (RMA) from the patient despite documenting the event in their patient care report. Their documentation did include whom they advised of the accident at the receiving facility.

As a result of this event, there is a management decision to standardize all the stretchers in the fleet. EMS practitioners are retrained on the operations of the critical care stretchers, and staff are in-serviced regarding the reporting requirements of such events.

Most negative outcome events are not the result of a single major failure but of a series of minor events that often go unnoticed until they reach a critical level that leads to an injury or other negative outcome.

WRAP-UP

Summary

- Crew resource management (CRM) is a tool originally instituted by the airline industry to optimize performance and outcomes by reducing the effect of human error through the use of all available resources. The goal of CRM training is to enable high-performance teams, such as airline or ambulance crews, to achieve and maintain collective situational awareness.

- When groups of competent, trained individuals get together to solve problems, they typically define the issue and then deploy a combination of "humanware," software, and hardware to solve the problem. The humanware component consists of those people who are part of a team and have been directed to solve a particular problem.

- EMS agencies with open communication and that embrace respectful and informed feedback as a method for encouraging collective situational awareness develop skills for their humanware to solve complex problems effectively within dynamic environments.

- Implementing the incident command system (ICS) is not a guarantee that the incident will be resolved flawlessly. CRM can highlight the areas where team communication breaks down and help EMS agencies to design specific strategies for improvement.

- Within high-performance teams, regular use of CRM continually improves performance. When teams practice communication techniques that are designed to share understanding, it provides opportunities to build team discipline, broaden the knowledge base of individual team members, and remove boundaries to learning. CRM can establish trust and respect within teams, reduce the chance for error caused by distraction, and encourage collective situational awareness.

- Most teams are created for a specific purpose—to get something done. The team leader needs to consider the number and types of objectives, their clarity, and their priority, with input from team members. Because often there are competing objectives and multiple methods for achieving them, effective leaders communicate what they perceive to be the priorities and then ask for input. Then they set a direction for the team.

- Situational awareness has three primary components: an awareness of the surroundings and how individuals are supposed to interact with the surroundings; the reality of the situation; and individual perceptions of the situation.

- Situational awareness is an internal active evaluation process that goes on constantly, much like size-up. EMS practitioners must update their situational awareness constantly by observing their surroundings, evaluating their options, and communicating with those around them.

- The typical CRM model contains several key elements, all of which are integral to gaining a shared understanding in a culture of learning and mutual respect. These elements are inquiry, advocacy, conflict resolution, decision, observe and critique, and discuss options.

- High-performance teams work best when they have a collective understanding of the situation that they face.

- Incident investigation finds that errors are not random in EMS. People cause accidents by making errors. Errors arise from poor communication, poor teamwork, and not paying attention. By mitigating errors, EMS practitioners can reduce deaths and injuries.

- There are personal strategies for error reduction. First, ensure a high level of proficiency in your knowledge and skills. Understand your policies and procedures. Have open communications and ensure that everyone on the team knows that he or she can call a safety time-out if things are not clear.

- Postincident analysis (PIA) is an activity that takes place after the incident to review the team's performance and the validity of current policies and focuses on identifying the lessons learned. The PIA is an opportunity to identify issues that may be occurring on a daily basis in order to prevent minor or major errors from occurring.

WRAP-UP (CONTINUED)

Glossary

challenge More direct than an alert; when a team member physically moves into the action circle, prepared to take the next step of emergency intervention.

coherence When truth aligns with some specified set of sentences, propositions, or beliefs.

conflict resolution A range of processes aimed at alleviating or eliminating sources of conflict; generally includes negotiation, mediation, and diplomacy.

crew resource management (CRM) A tool originally instituted by the airline industry in 1980 to optimize performance and outcomes by reducing the effect of human error through the use of all available resources.

hardware Solutions that take the form of computers, vehicles, tools, medications, or protective equipment.

high-reliability organizations (HROs) Organizations that operate in high-risk environments yet strive to maintain a learning atmosphere so as to minimize chances for error.

humanware The people who are part of a team that has been directed to solve a particular problem.

incident command system (ICS) A management tool that helps people manage emergency incidents by identifying incident needs and setting priorities.

postincident analysis (PIA) An activity involving team members that takes place after an incident response. It reviews performance of individuals and teams while focusing on learning lessons that can be applied to future incidents.

sense making The ability or attempt to make sense of an ambiguous situation.

situational awareness The state of being aware of what is happening to understand how information, events, and a person's actions will affect his or her goals and objectives, now and in the near future.

software Solutions that take the form of rewriting training materials or procedures or developing checklists or policies.

References

1. Baker D, Day R, Salas E. Teamwork as an essential component of high-reliability organizations. *Health Serv Res.* 2006; 41(4):1576–1598.

2. Heinrich HW. *Industrial Accident Prevention: A Scientific Approach.* New York, NY: McGraw-Hill; 1931.

Additional Readings

1. LeSage P, Dyar J, Evans B. *Crew Resource Management—Principles and Practice.* Burlington, MA: Jones & Bartlett Learning; 2011.
2. Bishop T. *Preventing Human Error Study Guide.* Payson, AZ: Error Prevention Institute; 2000.
3. Helmreich RL, Merritt AC. *Culture at Work in Aviation and Medicine.* Aldershot, UK: Ashgate Press; 1998.

4. Lubnau T II, Okray R. Crew resource management for the fire service. *Fire Engineering.* 2001;154(8). http://www.fireengineering.com/articles/print/volume-154/issue-8/features/crew-resource-management-for-the-fire-service.html. Accessed June 16, 2015.

CHAPTER 3

© Barbol/Shutterstock

Emergency Vehicle Safety

CHAPTER OBJECTIVES

After reading this chapter, the participant will be able to:

- Understand the risks associated with emergency vehicle operations

- Discuss risk-reducing driver behaviors

- Discuss the risks of excessive speed and the impact on the total stopping distance

- Describe the risks of operating in emergency mode

- Explore the impact of distracted driving

- Describe the concept of codriving

- Explain the importance of inspecting the ambulance and having preventive maintenance performed regularly

- Understand importance of securing EMS practitioners, patients, and equipment

- Describe the measures that can prevent injury in EMS practitioners who perform patient care while the ambulance is in motion

© Barbol/Shutterstock

SCENARIO

It's a normal night shift in the city. You and your partner have just picked up a regular patient complaining of abdominal pain. The patient is stable and is going for his weekly trip to his preferred hospital. As the emergency vehicle operator, you put on your seat belt before starting the ambulance. Your partner sits on the bench seat and alternates between attending to the patient on the stretcher and starting on the patient care report.

It's a nice clear evening, and you're cruising down a one-way street with the window down, watching the people on the sidewalk enjoying the summer night. Your phone is going off; your friends seem to be busy texting tonight.

All of a sudden, a car crosses into your lane. You yell, "Hold on!" and conduct a rapid lane change while hitting the brakes. Fortunately, the lane next to you is clear, and you manage to slow and avoid hitting the other car.

Unfortunately, your partner barely hears your warning. Your partner is unrestrained, and the rapid lane change and sudden deceleration cause your partner to fly head first into the wall dividing the cab and the patient compartment. You hear your partner hit the wall with a sickening thud. You call out your partner's name and hear no response.

You park the ambulance safely at the side of the road, activate the lights, and call for additional ambulances and staff cars. You enter the patient compartment and find your partner unresponsive. You immediately begin assessing your partner and hope for the best.

1. How can ambulances be made safer for EMS practitioners who are in the patient compartment?
2. What can be done to prevent injuries to patients and EMS practitioners in the patient compartment?
3. How can emergency vehicle operators stay focused on the road and not be distracted while driving the ambulance?

Introduction

This chapter is not intended to replace driver training; the goal of this chapter is to highlight the areas of emergency vehicle operations that too often cause injury and death. The National Association of Emergency Medical Technicians (NAEMT) and the EMS Safety Course Committee strongly recommend regular certified initial and refresher training for *all* emergency vehicle operators. This includes both a didactic course, with a focus on local policies, and a driver training course.

We live in a society that engages in many distractions while behind the wheel. In other words, too many drivers practice **aggressive driving**. These aggressive drivers are only worried about their own immediate needs, such as wanting to check a text message, and are not paying attention to what other drivers are doing or their own driving **FIGURE 3-1**. This is why it is critical that emergency vehicle operators are on the "defensive" at all times when on the road, especially when operating emergently. Emergency vehicle operators need to drive with due regard.

Many of the hazards of the road can be reduced or eliminated by safe driving practices. Additionally, emergency vehicle operators often have a partner in the cab who can help mitigate the risks of the road by operating as a team with the driver, as emphasized in Chapter 2: Crew Resource Management.

This chapter reviews the best practices for operating a vehicle safely. Many of these concepts may be familiar, but it is always good to review safe driving practices and integrate them into your everyday routine.

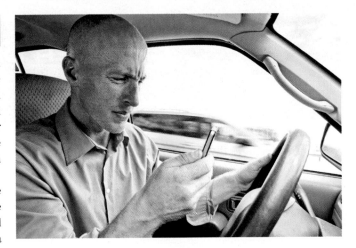

Figure 3-1 Aggressive drivers are only worried about their own immediate needs, such as wanting to check a text message, and are not paying attention to what other drivers are doing or to their own driving.

© becon/iStockphoto

Avoiding Collisions

Motor vehicle crashes (MVCs) involving ambulances are all too common and costly **FIGURE 3-2**. Approximately 10,000 MVCs occur each year, which damages EMS agencies' reputations and costs the agencies time, money, and personnel. These MVCs can cost the individuals involved their livelihoods, their health, and even their lives.

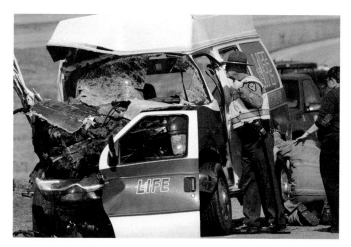

Figure 3-2 Motor vehicle crashes (MVCs) involving ambulances are all too common and costly.

© Frank Robertson/Chillicothe Gazette/AP Photo

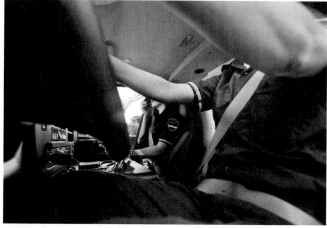

Figure 3-4 Seat belts save lives.

© Montgomery Martin/Alamy

EMS practitioners are more than 4 times more likely than the average worker to die in an MVC **FIGURE 3-3** .[1] To prevent deaths and increase safety for EMS practitioners, it is important to examine MVCs to identify the risks. By understanding the factors involved in MVCs, emergency vehicle operators can, it is hoped, avoid the risk factors and decrease the chances they will be involved in an MVC.

What the Data Say

The limited studies performed on MVCs involving ambulances show that a majority of the incidents occurred on days with no visibility issues and dry roads.[2] This means that many human factors are involved, as compared with weather and visibility problems. It should not be surprising that a majority of these MVCs occur in intersections with traffic signals in place. The most severe MVCs occur at intersections; however, head-on MVCs are the most deadly types of collisions.

The most important factor in the severity of an MVC is speed. Excessive speed is the most consistent factor in fatal MVCs involving ambulances. It is important to note that "excessive" is defined by the road, weather, and traffic conditions, not just by the posted speed limits. As vehicle speed increases, the driver's ability to react and respond decreases, just as the distance that is required to stop increases.

There are ways to decrease the chances of injury or death for EMS practitioners involved in MVCs. The first is to simply use properly the safety equipment provided in civilian and emergency vehicles. Seat belts save lives and increase the rates of survivability **FIGURE 3-4** . Because seat belts have been proved to save lives, it is critical to consistently wear them whenever possible, even when you are in the ambulance. We must find a way to work smarter while seat-belted when the ambulance is in motion **FIGURE 3-5** . Unfortunately, caring for a patient in the back of a moving ambulance does not grant you immunity from the laws of kinematics during an MVC.

EMS: an unsafe profession
Just how dangerous is it?

Transportation-related fatalities (per 100,000)

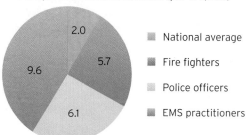

2.0
9.6
5.7
6.1

- National average
- Fire fighters
- Police officers
- EMS practitioners

Figure 3-3 A pie chart representing the number of transportation-related fatalities by profession.

Data from: Kahn, CA. EMS, first responders, and crash injury. *Top Emerg Med.* 2006;26:68–74.

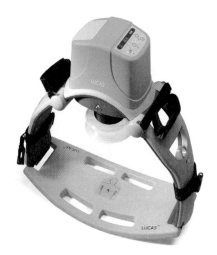

Figure 3-5 We must find a way to work smarter while seat-belted when the ambulance is in motion.

Courtesy of Physio-Control, Inc.

Personal Experience

As an EMS practitioner, it is important that you pay attention to any close calls that you have experienced personally. It is important to identify and study the conditions that led to any near misses. By identifying the risk factors, you can try to prevent them from happening again. For example, having a close call at a blind intersection may teach you to slow down and be careful at that intersection, keeping you from being involved in a future MVC at that location.

Examining your personal history is not the only way to learn from close calls, near misses, or MVCs. The EMS Voluntary Event Notification Tool (EVENT) is a system that all EMS practitioners should use. With EVENT, EMS practitioners can voluntarily and even anonymously report real events that have happened to them so that others can learn from their experiences. The information reported by EMS practitioners is collected in a database and analyzed. The analytics are used to help prevent similar events from occurring in the future through the development of preventive measures such as training programs and official policies. The collected data are sent on a quarterly and annual basis to state EMS offices and federal agencies with jurisdiction over the agencies. Those who have EMS affiliations are also able to sign up to see the reports. No individual responses are shared or transmitted to outside parties, such as the media. The EVENT reporting system is accessible through the NAEMT's website.

Risk Factors

The data on MVCs involving emergency vehicles show that four situations create the highest risks for collision. The most consistent risk factors are intersections, following distances, vehicle speed, and distraction. All EMS vehicle operators should obtain formal training in an Emergency Vehicle Operator (EVOC) course to improve skills and learn about the four risk factors in detail.

IN THE FIELD

Even during nonemergent driving, stopping at intersections can present challenges for emergency vehicle operators. The key is to leave room to "get out" when stopping at an intersection. The operator should stop and leave enough distance that the tires of the vehicle in front of the ambulance are visible against the pavement. This should allow for enough room for the ambulance to maneuver around the vehicle if it stalls or if there is an emergent run. The operator should always have a planned escape route.

IN THE FIELD

Most crashes are side impact and mirror-to-mirror because of the narrowing of lanes to accommodate bike lanes. On many roads, emergency vehicles are the same width as the traffic lanes, which does not leave room for steering or judgment errors.

Intersections

Intersections are where the most significant MVCs involving ambulances occur FIGURE 3-6 . Fortunately, there are preventive measures that emergency vehicle operators can take when approaching an intersection. As the emergency vehicle approaches the intersection, the emergency vehicle operator, or partner whenever possible, should change the siren's cadence. This will grab the attention of other drivers and alert them that the emergency vehicle is approaching. As the emergency vehicle enters the intersection, a secondary sound will also alert other drivers that an ambulance is near.

In any discussion on safety, it is important to mention that ambulances should stop at all controlled intersections. Each state, locality, and agency will have its own laws or policies that state exactly when emergency vehicles are required to stop at intersections. Even though it may be legal not to come to a complete stop, it is *highly* recommended that all ambulances come to a complete stop at controlled intersections while operating emergently. As the emergency vehicle enters the intersection, both the emergency vehicle operator and partner, when available, should be looking in both directions and clearing the intersection.

When at multi-lane intersections, it is important to slowly proceed through the intersection while clearing each lane. Also

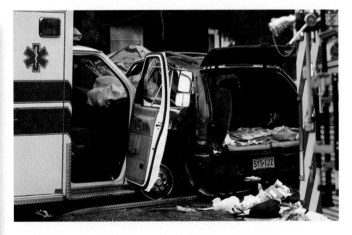

Figure 3-6 Intersections are where most MVCs involving ambulances occur.

remember not to push other vehicles into or through the intersection against the traffic signals.

Moving through controlled intersections against the signal presents a real danger to emergency vehicles and all others sharing the road. The same risk exists even in uncontrolled intersections and even when the ambulance has the right of way. It is important to watch your speed, slow down, change siren patterns, and even cover the brake with your foot in case a quick stop is required. Becoming complacent at any intersection can lead to an MVC.

Opticom and other similar signal control devices may be helpful in changing lights or keeping them green as your ambulance approaches. With these devices, it is important to pay attention for other emergency apparatus with signal control devices that are approaching the same intersection.

Finally, remember, the general rule with yellow lights is that they stay yellow for one second for every 10 miles per hour of the speed limit. This is why it is important to always be cautious and slow down when approaching an intersection and cover the brake with your foot.

Following Distance

Not allowing the proper stopping distance between the ambulance and the vehicle in front of it is another common cause of MVCs during both emergent and nonemergent driving. Ambulances are heavier than typical passenger vehicles, which means that these emergency vehicles require more distance to fully stop. Stopping and following distances also become an issue when multiple emergency vehicles are responding to the same incident. A police car can stop in a shorter distance than an ambulance, but an ambulance can stop in a shorter distance than a fire apparatus.

Many factors affect how long it takes to stop an ambulance. The brakes, speed, tires, and weather conditions all play a part in how quickly an ambulance can come to a stop. When ice, water, or other substances are on the road, the time and distance it takes to stop the ambulance will be increased. As a preventive measure, decrease your speed and increase your following distance during inclement weather. The same advice applies in areas of poor visibility or when there is a great need to make a sudden stop.

Another situation occurs when multiple emergency vehicles respond to the same scene. Multi-vehicle responses create significant hazards. If the vehicles are all traveling the same route, there must be enough space between the emergency vehicles for other drivers to see them and realize they must wait for more than one vehicle to pass. Using a separate and different siren cadence will also help alert drivers of the presence of a subsequent emergency vehicle.

Vehicle Speed

The speed of the ambulance will play a significant part in the operator's ability to avoid an MVC as well as the severity of the MVC should one occur. As mentioned, excessive speed is a common factor in fatal collisions. Excessive speed is not just based on the

---

IN THE FIELD

When traveling in traffic, the emergency vehicle operator should leave at least 4 seconds of following distance at speeds up to 40 miles per hour (mph) and then add at least one second for every 10 mph over 40 mph. The emergency vehicle operator should also look 12 seconds ahead to avoid potential hazards and traffic patterns. These are minimum recommendations. When weather or visibility issues exist, these following distances should be increased. The key is for operators to give themselves enough time to react and to give other drivers a chance to recognize the ambulance's intentions.

Whenever the emergency vehicle operator believes he or she is in an unsafe situation, it is paramount to try to find a way out and take extra precautions. If another driver is racing or tailgating, it is appropriate to move over and let the driver pass and create distance between the ambulance and the high-risk driver. One such situation may occur when a patient's family is following too close behind or chasing the ambulance. A quick discussion with the family before transport should prevent this situation altogether.

IN THE FIELD

The emergency vehicle operator should tell the patient's family members where the patient will be transported and that they should take their time and drive safely. The emergency vehicle operator should also tell the family that it will take a few minutes for the patient to be registered, assessed, and settled in a room, at which point they will be allowed to see the patient; therefore, they should take their time and drive safely to the facility.

---

posted speed limit but on the conditions of the roads. As speed increases, the distance traveled before a driver can see, react, and complete a defensive maneuver or stop increases. When weather factors such as ice, snow, or water on the road increase stopping distances and decrease visibility, emergency vehicle operators need to decrease their speed to below the posted speed limits to account for the increased stopping distances.

The kinetic energy of a potential collision is exponentially increased as the speed of the vehicle increases. This means that the force that impacts every object and person involved in a collision will increase significantly. These traumatic forces will travel into the ambulance and transfer to the emergency vehicle operator in the front, and the EMS practitioner and the patient in the back. Remember, if an EMS practitioner is unrestrained in the patient compartment, he or she will be traveling at the same speed as the ambulance until an outside force, such as a wall, suddenly collides against him or her. EMS practitioners working in ambulances involved in MVCs are subject to the same laws of kinematics and the same patterns of injuries as anyone else involved in an MVC. The biggest difference between civilian vehicle occupants and EMS practitioners is that EMS practitioners keep finding excuses not to be restrained while chastising their patients for the same behavior.

Distractions

The many distractions that can capture the emergency vehicle operator's attention while driving are covered in depth later in this chapter. The key point is to remember that driving is the primary responsibility of the emergency vehicle operator, and *everything else* can wait. The operator must be focused on driving the ambulance so that he or she is prepared to react and maneuver instantly to avoid MVCs. The first rule of coming into work is to go home from work safely. As the Crew Resource Management chapter discusses in detail, avoid the hazards of distractions by creating a "sterile cockpit" and utilize the principles of crew resource management to prevent MVCs.

The emergency vehicle operator also needs to know where he or she is going. Trying to navigate in unfamiliar areas can create a very serious distraction and cause the emergency vehicle operator to look around for street signs rather than pay attention to the road. Using the principles of crew resource management, the partner should act as a codriver and navigator so that the emergency vehicle operator can focus on driving. Ideally, the emergency vehicle operator should decide on a route before driving. GPS systems that "speak" may also help the emergency vehicle operator focus on the road instead of navigating. Training in navigation techniques using the numbering systems or coordinates is also helpful, but in the end, there is no substitute for having a good knowledge of the area.

IN THE FIELD

Remember to stay focused on the road and look for road hazards like potholes. Watch the crosswalk to avoid pedestrians who may not be aware of or acknowledge your rapidly approaching ambulance. Look ahead for changes in traffic patterns and signal changes. Emergency vehicle operators should be constantly preplanning and thinking about the "what-ifs" of driving, such as *What if a car pulled out in front of me?*

Backing

Operating in reverse, or backing, is one of the most dangerous maneuvers for an ambulance. Although operating in reverse most often occurs at lower speeds, backing is the cause of many incidents and collisions and even costs lives. According to the Department of Transportation (DOT), backing collisions account for 25% of all MVCs involving commercial vehicles. The DOT also reported that 18,000 injuries a year are due to backing. Finally, according to the DOT, about 292 fatalities occur each year from backing collisions.

IN THE FIELD

The children's advocacy group kidsandcars.org estimates that 50 children are seen in emergency rooms for accidents related to backing each week, and 2 children every week die from their injuries.

Considering that the average driver travels less than a mile a year in reverse, the injury and fatality data are staggering. There are several preventive actions that an emergency vehicle operator can take. First, do not disable the backing alarm on the ambulance. This is a warning device designed to alert people that the unit is backing and to stand clear. Even with cameras, there are blind spots when backing.

Use a spotter every time the ambulance operates in reverse to help decrease the chance of a collision **FIGURE 3-7**. EMS agencies should have policies that require spotters while backing even if backing cameras are present. If the view of the spotter is lost, the operator should stop the vehicle *immediately*. If the operator shifts his or her gaze from one mirror to another, he or she should stop the vehicle *immediately*. While it may

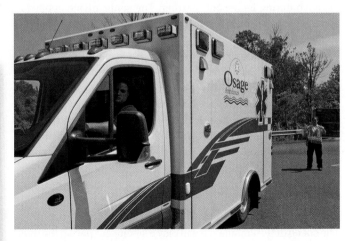

Figure 3-7   Use a spotter every time the ambulance backs to decrease the chance of a collision.

not always be possible to have a spotter outside the vehicle, if the EMS practitioner in the patient care compartment can watch at the back window, between the operator and the EMS practitioner, any blind spots may be covered without leaving the patient unattended.

Rate of Closure

Following distance and how fast an ambulance closes in on another vehicle can create dangerous situations. **Rate of closure** is the time it takes to close the distance between the ambulance and another vehicle, relative to the speeds of both vehicles. When you are driving in the emergent mode, it is important to allow other drivers to react to the presence of the ambulance. Drivers can be unpredictable when an emergency vehicle comes up behind them. Many times there is an initial panic on the part of the other driver, and he or she may try to stop or even turn into the path of the ambulance. If the ambulance is following too close or closing in too fast, this may result in an MVC. Emergency vehicle operators need to allow other drivers time to react and move out of the way. Emergency vehicle operators also need to leave enough room and slow their speeds so they can react to unpredictable drivers.

IN THE FIELD

- Leave yourself an escape route.
- Always maintain a safe following distance.
- Look ahead and watch traffic patterns.
- Give other drivers time to react to you.
- Use extreme caution if you are driving in tandem with another emergency vehicle.

It is important to know operationally pertinent local and state laws regarding emergency vehicles. Some states have changed from "move to the right" to "move to the closest curb." This is helpful on larger roads, especially one-way streets. Because the law varies from state to state, drivers may follow the law of the state in which they first learned to drive and not the law of the state they are currently driving in. Never expect a driver to move a certain way. Be prepared to react to unpredictable drivers by leaving enough following distance and not closing in on other vehicles so rapidly that you surprise the drivers.

Speed

Speed reduces a driver's ability to react and increases the potential traumatic consequences. As discussed, speed reduces the emergency vehicle operator's ability to react quickly while exposing the occupants of the ambulance to increased levels of trauma. An emergency vehicle operator who presses his or her foot down on the accelerator chooses to speed despite the knowledge of its potential consequences. Every EMS practitioner is taught that speed exponentially increases the kinetic energy that occurs during a collision and that by speeding, the chance of injury in the event of a collision increases. This violates the vow "first, do no harm."

Acceleration and speed can quickly get an emergency vehicle operator away from a potentially dangerous situation, but continuous speeding is dangerous because speed is a contributing factor in an average of 30% of all fatal crashes per year, according to the National Highway Traffic Safety Administration (NHTSA). The reason used to justify speeding by many operators is the need to reach patients quickly. However, several studies have shown that speeding during emergent driving saves very little time and only makes a difference in very few patient care situations.[3,4]

Some emergency vehicle operators have shown **siren syndrome**, in which an emergency vehicle operator begins to drive aggressively when the siren switches on. With siren syndrome, the emergency vehicle operator believes that all other drivers should hear the ambulance's siren, and the right-of-way should be handed over immediately. Increased adrenaline leads to disregarding the conditions of the road and practicing dangerous maneuvers. Training and practicing on closed courses in emergent mode with sirens on and educating emergency vehicle operators about siren syndrome can help prevent this dangerous occurrence.[5]

IN THE FIELD

The key term in most states is **due regard**, which is the idea that the operator driving in the emergency mode should give regard and attention to everyone else sharing the road.

Many EMS agencies believe that it is important to have clearly labeled policies that limit how fast ambulances can travel. It is important to remember that if your agency's policies restrict the speed of the ambulance, the policy may carry the weight of law in your state and can add increased legal liability.

Total Stopping Distance

Stopping a moving vehicle is a multi-step process. The steps are the same no matter which mode the ambulance is operating in, but when the vehicle's speed increases, so does the distance traveled at each step. The first step of stopping is the time it takes to recognize that the ambulance needs to stop, which is called **human perception time**. **Human reaction time** is the second step, which is the time it takes the emergency vehicle operator to actually cover the brake pedal with his or her foot and press down.

The next two steps, **vehicle reaction time** and **vehicle braking time**, are not controlled by the emergency vehicle operator but rely on the vehicle to respond the way it is supposed to. In many cases, stopping depends on the vehicle being properly maintained. The brakes have to activate, grab, and create friction to slow the vehicle. If the emergency vehicle operator is driving with the brake pedal covered (two-footed driving) or if the brakes have been heavily used, this may be difficult. The tires also have to actually grab the road. When water, ice, or other slick substances are on the road, traction between the road and the tires may be compromised. Tire pressure and tread wear will also impact the traction, which is why it is critical that the emergency vehicle operator ensure that the ambulance is ready for the road.

It is important to remember that these numbers apply to the average vehicle on the road, not something as heavy as a fully loaded ambulance. Based on the type and weight, the ambulance's stopping distance will actually be longer.

Emergency Driving

There are many terms for operating an ambulance in the emergency mode, including running hot, code 3 driving, or using lights and sirens. Operating in the emergency mode is a significant factor in ambulance collisions **FIGURE 3-8**. According to the NHTSA, 70% of ambulance collisions occur while using lights and sirens. With so many collisions attributed to emergent operations, the obvious answer seems to be to reduce operating emergently. Studies show that using lights and sirens does not save much time during transport, causes more stress, and is dangerous for ambulance crews.[3,4] When operating emergently, everyone is at risk, and it is harder to perform patient care. A strong emergency medical dispatch (EMD) program can help limit emergency responses by clinically determining who needs an emergent response for a potentially life-threatening illness or injury versus who can wait longer for an ambulance. Then a strong protocol-based clinical judgment will help decrease emergency transports to hospitals by limiting emergency transports to unstable, life-threatening situations.

IN THE FIELD

Remember that the level of experience and skill among drivers differs greatly. Ambulances share the road with variable skill, experience, and reaction times.

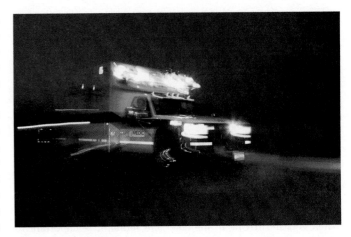

Figure 3-8 Operating in the emergency mode is a significant factor in ambulance collisions.
© Stockbyte/Thinkstock

Think back to your last emergent transport to the hospital. Were you able to work and attend to the needs of the patient? Was the ride smoother than a nonemergent transport? Did the patient's anxiety increase? Finally, did the public quickly and properly move out of the way? In many cases, emergent driving is not very smooth because the public reacts unpredictably to lights and sirens. This can cause issues with patient care and increases the chance of injury to the EMS practitioner working in the back. Also, the patient may experience increased anxiety from a rough ride, which could make conditions such as heart attacks worse.

Distractions

Distractions increase the risk of collisions. Driving distractions include music, conversation, sightseeing, cell phones, mobile data terminals, GPS, and food. All these distractions can be controlled. To prevent MVCs due to distractions, EMS needs to adopt the principles of crew resource management and create a sterile cab. Distractions need to be reduced to only the most necessary of equipment.

Visual distractions are anything that lures you to take your eyes off the road. This type of distraction can be caused by coworkers pointing out sights along the side of the road, or a GPS map that an emergency vehicle operator is trying to use for navigation. Even the mobile data computer (MDC) with new run information can create a visual distraction for the operator.

Manual distractions cause you to take your hands off the wheel **FIGURE 3-9**. There are several overlaps between visual and manual distractions. For example, when an emergency vehicle operator reaches for an item, he or she will first look to see where the item is and then take one hand off the wheel to reach for the item. Items such as siren switches and radios are manual distractions. Even marking status changes with an MDC causes the operator to remove a hand from the wheel and is a manual distraction.

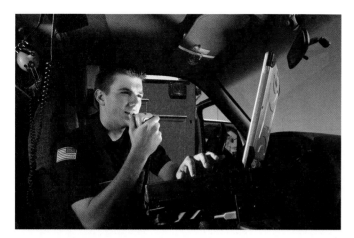

Figure 3-9 Visual and manual distractions can overlap and cause you to take your eyes off of the road and hands off of the wheel.

© Bounce/Cultura/Getty

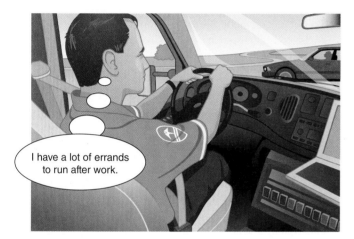

I have a lot of errands to run after work.

Figure 3-10 A cognitive distraction is anything that takes your mind off operating the vehicle.

© Jones & Bartlett Learning.

Cognitive distractions take your mind off the road **FIGURE 3-10**. Cognitive distractions can be both run related and non-run related. To avoid cognitive distractions, it is important to stop personal conversations when driving in the ambulance. Talking is not forbidden, but it should be related to the road, the scene, and safely arriving at the destination. Cognitive distractions are not just related to conversations; they can be personal issues that are distracting the operator. The emergency vehicle operator should be focused on driving, not what's for dinner, an argument with a significant other, or anything besides the task at hand.

Text Messaging

Texting is a "perfect storm." It requires you to:

1. Look at the screen and read a message (visual)
2. Manually manipulate the keys to write a message (manual)
3. Think about what you are writing (cognitive)

This means texting is a visual, manual, and cognitive distraction all in one. Texting while driving is also an example of a self-reinforcing behavior. Drivers get away with it repeatedly, which reinforces the behavior. But the reality is that emergency vehicle operators are unable to adhere to the responsibility of driving an ambulance with utmost caution while engaged in this highly dangerous practice. Data from the Virginia Tech Transportation Institute show that texting increases the risk of being in an MVC or near-MVC by 23.2 times. How many MVCs have you responded to because of texting?

Many states have noticed that mobile communication devices such as cell phones have led to increased MVCs. Several states have taken the approach of banning these devices at various levels. Some states limit texting and emailing while driving; other states have banned all devices without hands-free operation. A few states have attempted to ban all phone use while driving to eliminate distracted drivers.

Unfortunately, cellular devices are not the only type of distraction that increases MVCs. See **TABLE 3-1** for a list of various driver distractions and how much they increase the chance of an MVC.

Codriving

Following the principles of crew resource management will help the ambulance crew to share the responsibility of safe driving on the way to a call. Partners should be communicating, double-checking intersections, and alerting each other to potential road hazards **FIGURE 3-11**. The person in the driver's seat needs to focus on operating the vehicle. When there is a codriver in the passenger seat, that person should be responsible for siren changes, navigating, responding to the radio or MDC, and any other nondriving task that needs to be performed en route. During patient transport, the emergency vehicle operator will have to perform all these tasks. Limiting emergent

Table 3-1 Common Driving Distractions	
	Increased Risk (Times)
Drinking (Nonalcoholic)	Even
Eating	1.6
Applying Makeup	3.1
Drinking (Alcoholic)	4.1
Reaching for Moving Object	8.8
Texting	**23.2**

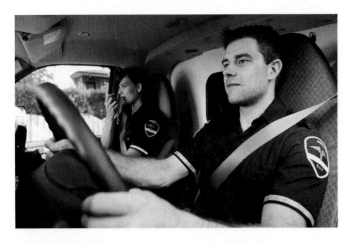

Figure 3-11 The person in the driver's seat needs to focus solely on operating the vehicle.

© Tyler Olson/Shutterstock

STAY IN THE FIELD

Talk and look before you move.

transport is key to decreasing the times when a codriver is not there to help.

Codrivers can be considered a distraction—but a protective distraction, because a cooperative partner can reduce the risks of driving emergently by staying engaged as a codriver.

It is important that both parties know their roles, depending on which position they occupy. EMS agencies should implement polices that clearly define the roles of personnel on the way to a run. When clear policies are put in place, EMS practitioners will function in the same manner and have the same roles no matter who is paired together.

Distracted Driving
Habits Need to Change

See TABLE 3-2 for a list of 10 things you can do today to personally combat distracted driving.

Don't forget that other drivers may be distracted. Stay alert, and stay away from those who are blinded by distraction! There is room for EMS personnel and services to create programs to reduce distracted driving not only within EMS agencies but also in the communities in which they serve. On scene immediately following a collision is not the time to educate the public about distracted driving; it is important to find a way to change the culture in the community at large and make the roads safer for *everyone.*

Table 3-2 **Combat Distracted Driving**
1. Leave your phone on silent and out of reach, and only check for messages when your vehicle has been placed in park.
2. Have your partner answer your phone or reply for you.
3. If you need to have a phone conversation or text, have your partner drive.
4. Secure all objects.
5. Have your partner navigate or plan your route before driving.
6. Have your partner handle the radios when possible.
7. Talk on the radio only when it is safe to do so—that is, before placing the vehicle in drive, at red lights, etc.
8. Place out of sight and reach any object that you feel may distract you.
9. Pull over to the side of the road if you feel the need to deviate from a safe practice.
10. Get a good night's sleep, and don't drive while drowsy (sleep is discussed in detail in Chapter 7: Personal Health).

Vehicle Inspections and Maintenance
Vehicle Inspections

Ambulances are poorly designed for maneuverability, quick stops, and handling under excessive forces. Because of this, a well-maintained and routinely inspected vehicle is a crucial component of ambulance safety. Vehicle inspections should be taught, monitored, documented, and retained FIGURE 3-12. Each EMS agency will have its own policies and procedures on what it expects ambulance crews to do in a daily vehicle check. There should be a formalized list of items that, if present, indicate the ambulance should be taken out of service immediately. If crews believe that a vehicle is unsafe, they should be able to take the ambulance out of service until it is repaired. Crews also have the responsibility to report all minor issues before they become larger issues.

Vehicle Maintenance

All the people and equipment that help EMS practitioners do their jobs safely should be respected, particularly vehicles. EMS practitioners should get to know their fleet mechanics; it will help both the EMS practitioners and the fleet mechanics to develop respect for each other's challenges. The fleet mechanics can teach ambulance crews about the specifics of the vehicle and share the warning signs that indicate a potential issue. If there is a strong relationship between the ambulance crew and fleet mechanics, the fleet mechanics will be more apt to listen to the ambulance crew and investigate complaints about and issues with the ambulance.

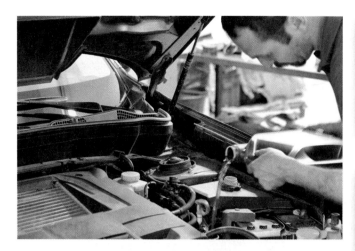

Figure 3-12 Vehicle inspections are a crucial component in preventing MVCs.
© LeventKonuk/iStockphoto

Respect Your Vehicles

Without the ambulance, patients will not be transported to the hospital. In many cases, the ambulance is the home of the ambulance crew during every shift. For these reasons alone, it is important to have respect for the ambulance. It is a very expensive and complicated piece of machinery. If emergency vehicle operators take care of their equipment, their equipment should function correctly and serve the entire ambulance crew and patients well. Ignoring minor issues, delaying repairs, and "pencil whipping" the inspection sheet will lead to many problems with the ambulance. If the ambulance breaks down during a call, patient care will suffer, and the disabled ambulance may become involved in an MVC.

Everyone and Everything Restrained

The risk of occupational injury and death is disproportionately high for EMS personnel, and the majority of casualties are associated with transportation incidents. Simply put, ambulances are not built or used in the same manner as standard passenger vehicles, resulting in safety concerns for both EMS practitioners and patients. Although there are inherent risks to occupants in an ambulance, some of the vulnerabilities can be reduced by properly restraining the occupants and equipment.

Seat Belt Use

Seat belts should be used by everyone, every time. The emergency vehicle operator should *never* be without a seat belt. In addition, any occupants in the ambulance should be properly restrained, including the patient and, if possible, those attending to the patient. Seat belts save lives, and there is *no* excuse for not wearing them in the passenger compartment. Seat belt indicator lights and alarms should *not* be deactivated.

STAY IN THE FIELD

Seat belts need to be used every time. There is no excuse for emergency vehicle operators and EMS practitioners not to be restrained.

STAY IN THE FIELD

Surveys show that a small percentage of EMS personnel *still* do not routinely use seat belts in the cab! Emergency or not, everyone should always use seat belts while in motion. Remember, most EMS agency policies require restraint use.[6] Emergency vehicle operators should take responsibility for ensuring occupant restraint use.[7]

Patient Compartment

Failure to use the provided restraint systems creates risks for all occupants, whether personally restrained or not. EMS practitioners and patients can become projectiles, endangering themselves and others FIGURE 3-13 . There is an increased vulnerability in the patient care compartment and risks to EMS practitioners and patients based on this factor.

The design of the ambulance and the nature of working in a moving vehicle make simply being in the patient compartment dangerous. In addition, the structure and the positions of ambulance seats in the patient compartment are dangerous.

Injuries can happen in the patient care compartment without an actual collision. Sudden evasive maneuvers, curb strikes, aggressive braking, unanticipated cornering, and slips/falls can all injure ambulance crew members attending to patients. The ambulance crew can fall on patients, into the walls, or even into the front cab if the emergency vehicle operator makes a sudden maneuver.

Occupants in traditional cardiopulmonary resuscitation (CPR) seat configurations in patient care compartments have been shown in numerous tests to experience a high likelihood of severe injury during frontal impact/frontal deceleration events.[8,9] The seat is not properly protected and often sits up against shelves without providing enough proper padding to protect the occupant. In addition, the EMS practitioner's head and spine are also at risk during side impacts. Unlike a car seat that a child uses, these CPR seats have no head and neck protection for a head-on collision.

All equipment must be completely secured or tied down. Monitors, patient report computers, and other unsecured equipment become missiles during MVCs or sudden evasive

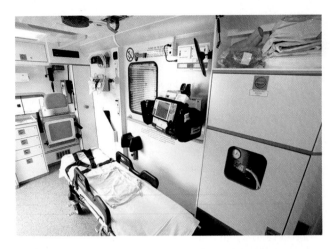

Figure 3-13 Secure all potential projectiles in the patient care compartment.

© Jones & Bartlett Learning

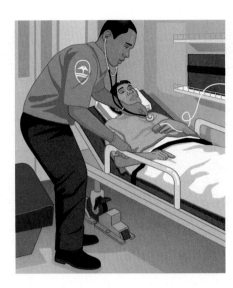

Figure 3-14 If you must be unrestrained and moving in the patient compartment during transport, it is imperative that you maintain three points of contact with the ambulance.

© Jones & Bartlett Learning.

maneuvers. All cabinets should be locked and stay closed. In the event of an MVC or sudden stop, unlocked cabinets can release their items and injure both EMS practitioners and patients.

Risk Mitigation

Avoid Injury

One key to reducing injury is to use proper restraints whenever possible, including in the patient care compartment. The rear-facing jump seat or airway seat is the preferred place to sit when possible. Avoid standing when the ambulance is in motion. Standing leads to more risk for everyone in the patient care compartment because if an EMS practitioner falls, he or she could injure the patient or fellow ambulance crew member. If the EMS practitioner feels that he or she must be unrestrained and moving in the patient compartment during transport, it is imperative that the EMS practitioner maintain three points of contact with the ambulance **FIGURE 3-14**. Balancing or "surfing" with only the EMS practitioner's feet on the ground will do nothing to protect the EMS practitioner from being thrown during a sudden maneuver or collision.

Decreasing the number of people in the patient care compartment will also reduce the risk of injury. Do not take more people than is absolutely necessary.

Finally, using technology to automate some aspects of patient care may allow EMS practitioners to spend more time restrained in their seats. The more hands-off patient care can be during transportation, the less risk of injury.

Working in Motion

Preparation and Ergonomics Actions

Making ambulances safer will take time, new standards, and considerable cost. As new designs and standards emerge,

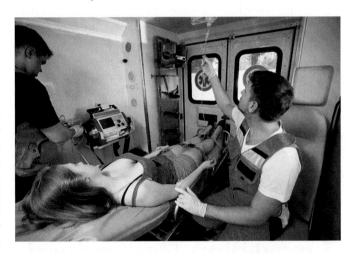

Figure 3-15 Try to place patient care report computers and monitors in mounts where they are secure and within reach.

© Photographee.eu/Shutterstock

ambulances will be safer. In the meantime, actions can be taken now to improve ambulance safety—for example, having machines that automatically take the patient's vitals so that EMS practitioners can remain seated and secured with a seat belt while monitoring the patient. Before loading the patient into the ambulance, when it is medically possible, take a few minutes at the scene to perform such procedures as starting and securing intravenous equipment (IVs) before leaving so that EMS practitioners can be seated during transport.

Try to place patient care report computers and monitors in mounts where they are secure and within reach of a restrained EMS practitioner **FIGURE 3-15**. Remember that emergency driving with unrestrained occupants in the patient care compartment can lead to serious injury and must be avoided.

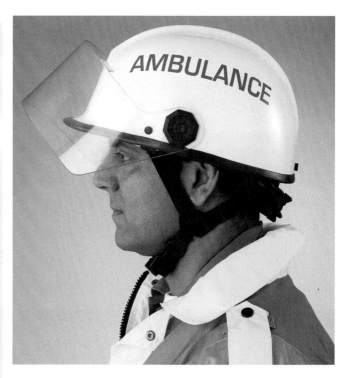

Figure 3-16 Helmets could increase safety for EMS practitioners on scene and during transport.

© Volt Collection/Shutterstock

Helmets

There is a trend to outfit ambulance crews with helmets **FIGURE 3-16**. These helmets could increase safety on scene and during transport. European and Australian ambulance services require that lightweight helmets be worn in the patient care compartment. With some studies showing that around 65% of fatal accidents involve head injury, it is important to examine the potential injury reduction a helmet could add.[10]

To be helpful, the helmet would have to be lightweight and not have any tails or protrusions that could cause a neck injury in a collision. The National Fire Protection Association's standard NFPA 1901: Standard for Automotive Fire Apparatus states that structural firefighting helmets are not to be used in vehicles because of their shape and weight. It is also important that the helmet not limit the vision of the emergency vehicle operator.

It is worth examining the benefits of helmet use given that our goal is to do whatever possible to decrease injuries and deaths of EMS practitioners. It will take a change in the culture of EMS, but if EMS practitioners see that helmets can save lives, they should be willing to accept the change.

Transporting Patients
Adults

It is hard to find a position that is perfectly safe for all patients in all situations. The main job of EMS is to transfer patients, but doing this perfectly safely may be difficult. The stretcher is the most common and proper place for the patient to sit. Of course, the assumption is that the stretcher is properly attached and secured to the ambulance. The other key is to use all the sets of straps that the manufacturer recommends and with the proper metal ends. In the ideal situation, the patient will be sitting with all the straps on, facing the rear of the ambulance, but this depends on the patient's condition.

Pediatric Challenges

Children present a unique set of challenges. The stretcher is made for adult weights and sizes, not for pediatric patients.

Proper child restraint safety systems are based on the child's weight and size. Ideally, a pediatric patient restraint system should adapt to various sizes of children to successfully and properly restrain them.

Children can become upset when removed from caregivers. However, parents should *never* be allowed to hold a child during transport because the child will not be restrained in a parent's arms.

IN THE FIELD

According to EMS for Children (EMSC) experts, we should:
- Use properly sized child restraint devices.
- Fully secure child restraint systems per the manufacturer's guidelines.
- Ensure that *all* occupants are restrained when the ambulance is in motion.
  In addition, according to EMSC experts:
  - We should *not* transport children who are not patients.
    - Use alternate transportation in a passenger vehicle when available.

- Do *not* allow parents, caregivers, EMS practitioners, or other passengers to be unrestrained during transport.
- Do *not* have the child/infant held in the parent's, caregiver's, or EMS practitioner's arms or lap during transport.
- The stretcher alone is not a restraint system for the pediatric patient.

WRAP-UP

Summary

- The ambulance is the only piece of equipment that is used on every call, yet EMS spends the least amount of time acquiring, assessing, and maintaining proficiency.
- Because too many drivers practice aggressive driving, emergency vehicle operators need to drive with due regard and drive with concern for others on and around the roadway.
- Many of the hazards of the road can be reduced or eliminated by safe driving practices.
- Approximately 10,000 MVCs occur each year, which costs EMS agencies time, money, and personnel. These MVCs can cost the individuals involved their livelihoods, their health, and even their lives.
- The EMS Voluntary Event Notification Tool (EVENT) is a system that all EMS practitioners should use. With EVENT, EMS practitioners can voluntarily and even anonymously report real events that have happened to them so that others can learn from their experiences.
- The data on MVCs involving emergency vehicles show that four situations create the highest risks for collision. The most consistent risk factors are intersections, following distances, vehicle speed, and distractions.
- The emergency vehicle operator can take preventive measures at intersections, including changing the siren's cadence, stopping at all controlled intersections, and stopping and clearing each lane of travel in multi-lane intersections. Becoming complacent at any intersection can lead to an MVC.

- Following distance and how fast an ambulance closes in on another vehicle can create dangerous situations. When driving in the emergent mode, it is important to allow other drivers to react to the presence of the ambulance.
- The speed of the ambulance will play a significant role in the emergency vehicle operator's ability to avoid an MVC as well as the severity of the MVC should one occur. As speed increases, the distance traveled before a driver can see, react, and complete a defensive maneuver or stop increases.
- Distractions increase the risk of collisions. Distractions need to be reduced to only the most necessary equipment.
  - Visual distractions are anything that lures you to take your eyes off the road.
  - Manual distractions are things that cause you to take your hands off the wheel.
  - Cognitive distractions are things that take your mind off the road.
- Texting is a perfect storm of distractions. It requires you to look at the screen and read a message, manually manipulate the keys to write a message, and think about what you are writing. This means that texting is a visual, manual, and cognitive distraction all in one.
- Data from the Virginia Tech Transportation Institute show that texting increases the risk of being in an MVC or near-MVC 23.2 times.
- Operating in reverse or backing is one of the most dangerous maneuvers for an ambulance. There are several

WRAP-UP (CONTINUED)

- preventive actions that an emergency vehicle operator can take, including activating the backing alarm on the ambulance and using a spotter every time the ambulance operates in reverse.
- Stopping a moving vehicle is a multi-step process. The steps are the same no matter which mode the ambulance is operating in, but when the vehicle's speed increases, so does the distance traveled at each step.
- Operating in the emergency mode is a significant factor in ambulance collisions. According to the NHTSA, 70% of ambulance collisions occur while operating emergently. One solution may be to reduce the amount of time operating emergently.
- Following the principles of crew resource management will help the ambulance crew to share the responsibility of safe driving on the way to a call. Partners should be communicating, double-checking intersections, and alerting each other to potential road hazards.

- Emergency vehicle operators should plan their routes before driving. Partners should be used to help navigate to the scene whenever possible.
- A well-maintained and routinely inspected vehicle is a crucial component of ambulance safety. Vehicle inspections should be taught, monitored, documented, and retained.
- Seat belts should be used by everyone, every time. The emergency vehicle operator should *never* be without a seat belt. In addition, any occupants in the ambulance should be properly restrained, including the patient and, if possible, those attending to the patient.
  - If an EMS practitioner must be unrestrained in the patient compartment while the ambulance is in motion, he or she must make sure to keep three points of contact with the ambulance.
- All equipment needs to be completely secured or tied down. Monitors, patient report computers, and other unsecured equipment become missiles during MVCs or sudden evasive maneuvers. All cabinets should be locked and stay closed.

Glossary

aggressive driving Operating a vehicle with aggressive actions, without concern for other drivers.

cognitive distractions Distractions that take the emergency vehicle operator's mind off the road and operation of the vehicle.

due regard When driving in emergency mode, the emergency vehicle operator should give regard and attention to everyone else sharing the road.

human perception time The time it takes a person to realize that he or she needs to react to an impending event.

human reaction time The time it takes for a person to react to an impending event.

manual distractions Distractions that cause the emergency vehicle operator to take a hand off the ambulance wheel.

rate of closure The speed at which a vehicle overtakes another.

siren syndrome When an emergency vehicle operator begins to drive aggressively and without regard for the conditions of the road during emergent operations.

vehicle braking time The time it takes for the vehicle to stop.

vehicle reaction time The time between when the brake pedal is applied and when the brakes start working.

visual distractions Distractions that take the emergency vehicle operator's eyes off the road.

References

1. Kahn C. EMS, first responders, and crash injury. *Top Emerg Med*. 2006;26:68–74.
2. Elling R. Dispelling myths on ambulance accidents. *JEMS*. 1989;14(7):60–64.
3. Brown L, Hunt R, Whitney C, Addario M, Hogue T. Do warning lights and sirens reduce ambulance response times? *Prehosp Emerg Care*. 2000;4(1):70–74.
4. Hunt R, Brown L, Cabinum E, Whitley T, Prasad N, Owens C Jr, Mayo C. Is ambulance transport time with lights and sirens faster than that without? *Ann Emerg Med*. 1995;25(4):507–511.
5. U.S. Fire Administration. Emergency Vehicle Safety Initiative. U.S. Department of Homeland Security. Washington DC. 2014. https://www.usfa.fema.gov/downloads/pdf/publications/fa_336 .pdf. Accessed April 26, 2015.

WRAP-UP (CONTINUED)

6. Auerbach P, Morris J Jr, Phillips J Jr, Redlinger S, Vaughn W. An analysis of ambulance accidents in Tennessee. *JAMA*. 1987;258(11):1487–1490.

7. Beckera LR, Zaloshnjaa E, Levickb N, Lic G, Millera T. Relative risk of injury and death in ambulances and other emergency vehicles. *ScienceDirect*. 2003;35(6):941–948.

8. Hui-Chih Wang, Wen-Chu Chiang, Shey-Ying Chen, et al. Video-recording and time-motion analyses of manual versus mechanical cardiopulmonary resuscitation during ambulance transport. *Resuscitation*. 2007;74(3):453–460.

9. Olaveengen T, Wik L, Steen P. Quality of cardiopulmonary resuscitation before and during transport in out-of-hospital cardiac arrest. *Resuscitation*. 2008;76(2):185–190.

10. Levick NR, Garigan M. A solution to head injury protection for emergency medical service providers. http://www.objective-safety.net/LevickIEA2006.pdf. Accessed June 15, 2015.

Additional Readings

1. Turner DJ. RETT mobile and the future of EMS safety. *EMS World*. August 1, 2013. http://www.emsworld.com/article/10978797/ambulance-and-ems-safety-innovations-from-europe. Accessed June 15, 2015.

2. Custalow CB, Gravitz CS. Emergency medical vehicle collisions and potential for preventive intervention. *Prehosp Emerg Care*. 2004;8(2):175–184.

3. National Highway Traffic Safety Administration. Working Group Best Practice Recommendations for the Safe Transportation of Children in Emergency Ground Ambulances. Washington DC. 2012.

Responsibilities in Roadway Operations

CHAPTER OBJECTIVES

After reading this chapter, the participant will be able to:

- Understand the risks to EMS practitioners during highway incidents

- Discuss the methods that EMS practitioners can use to protect themselves during roadway operations

© Barbol/Shutterstock

SCENARIO

It's a bright summer afternoon when you and your partner respond to a motor vehicle crash (MVC). As you arrive on scene, you find a downed motorcycle wedged underneath an SUV and a patient lying in the road. You park the ambulance as quickly as possible, and you and your partner walk quickly to tend to the victim. You reach the victim and find that his chest is not rising. You and your partner remove his helmet and begin ventilations. As you are getting your immobilization equipment in place and your partner is ventilating the patient with a bag-mask device, a car swerves toward you. You yell a warning and leap out of the way. You hear a crash, and when you look up, you see your partner pinned between a sedan and the SUV.

1. How should the ambulance be positioned at a motor vehicle crash?
2. What is your first priority at the scene?
3. What is your next action?

Introduction

Every day, emergency medical services (EMS) practitioners put themselves in harm's way when they respond to incidents on busy roads and highways throughout the country. While there to provide care for ill and injured patients, EMS practitioners too often become victims themselves when distracted drivers fail to see them and strike them with their vehicles. Roadway operations pose significant risks to EMS practitioners and other responders, as well as to patients and bystanders **FIGURE 4-1**.

Over the years, both the federal government and individual states have enacted laws in an effort to curb injuries and death to emergency personnel responding to incidents on roadways. Currently 49 states have some type of "Move Over or Slow Down" law in place to protect emergency responders and highway workers. Additionally, national campaigns like "Move Over, America" have taken up the cause to try to educate drivers on what to do when they approach emergency workers operating on a roadway.

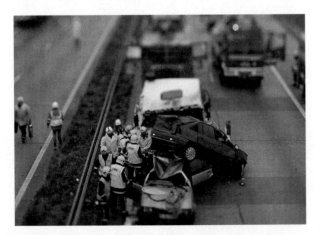

Figure 4-1 Roadway operations are a significant safety risk to EMS practitioners and other responders, as well as to patients and bystanders.

© Walter Bibikow/Photolibrary/Getty

Cultural changes throughout society are needed for safe operations on the roadways. In addition, all emergency responders need to work together in our approach and management of roadway incidents to improve scene safety for all. This includes changing our individual beliefs from "It can't happen to me" to "What can I do to prevent it from happening to me?" We need to understand local protocols and response plans, use all available safety equipment, have the right attitude about safety, and work with other emergency response agencies so we know what resources will be available to us on the road.

The Dangers of the Road

Responding to roadside incidents is dangerous for all emergency responders. The statistics speak for themselves:

- According to the National Law Enforcement Officers Memorial, 12 law enforcement officers are killed after being struck by vehicles at roadside incidents annually.
- According to the National Fallen Firefighters Memorial, five fighters are killed while responding to roadside incidents annually.
- According to the International Towing and Recovery Hall of Fame and Museum, 60 tow operators are killed while responding to roadside incidents annually.

Unfortunately, there is no central point of data collection to determine the number of EMS practitioners killed while responding to roadside incidents. Additionally, finding the numbers of EMS practitioners who are injured is extremely difficult because in many cases, these numbers are not tracked. Add to this the number of near misses that are never reported, and you have a very large number of EMS practitioners who are killed, injured, or almost injured when responding to roadside incidents.

According to the National Highway Traffic Safety Administration, on average, 10 crashes occur every minute that result in injuries in the United States. If we were to assume that each collision requires the response of two law enforcement officers, four fire fighters, two EMS practitioners, and one tow truck operator, that puts nine emergency response personnel at the scene at each MVC.[1] If we expand our view, we see:

- 90 emergency responders arriving at MVCs every minute
- 5,400 emergency responders working at MVCs every hour
- 130,000 emergency responders in a 24-hour period exposed to traffic hazards while working at an MVC

Because of the sheer volume of roadside incidents, it is critical that all emergency responders and EMS practitioners take proactive safety measures before the incident, when arriving at the incident, and when operating at the incident.

Preplanning for Safety
Traffic Incident Management Plans

Because we cannot control every variable every time while operating on a roadway, every possible safety precaution must be taken to increase our safety. To do this, every agency should have or participate in the creation of a **Traffic Incident Management (TIM)** plan. A TIM plan is a preplanning document created with the input of all emergency responding agencies, from law enforcement to fire to EMS to towing. A TIM plan ensures that all agencies will work together to secure the scene, maintain scene safety, care for and safely extract patients from the scene, and clear the scene as efficiently and safely as possible.[2] The TIM plan should spell out the roles and responsibilities of each agency, arrival procedures, and operating procedures. The goal is that every agency and emergency responder will be operating from the same page and with the safety of all emergency responders, patients, and bystanders in mind.

Vehicle Visibility

Visibility of emergency vehicles is important to emergency responders, but even more important to the general public. You may think, "How can the public not see emergency vehicles when they are lit up like a Christmas tree?" In 2009, the Federal Emergency Management Association (FEMA) released a study, the Emergency Vehicle Visibility and Conspicuity Study (FA-323), on the importance of enhancing vehicle visibility using conspicuity products. **Conspicuity** is the ability of a vehicle to draw the attention of other drivers. Enhancing a vehicle's conspicuity is not just about making it easily visible but also about enhancing the safety of the emergency vehicle and the public. Various factors affect the visibility of an ambulance, including size, color scheme, and emergency lighting.

Studies have shown that flashing lights, versus steady, are far superior for gaining attention of other drivers.[3] A combination of red and yellow colors in the flashing lights package has proved to be popular as a warning and caution identifier. The red and yellow are used because they signify "danger."

Research suggests that color, patterns, and reflectivity will make emergency vehicles more visible and help to reduce the incidence of other drivers crashing into ambulances.[4] The use of contrasting fluorescent colors and reflective colors has been shown to assist drivers in locating hazards on the roadway, both day and night.[4] Creating patterns to be placed on the ambulance using contrasting fluorescent colors increases the conspicuity of the vehicle. Since 2000, the United Kingdom has used the Battenburg pattern, alternating contrasting fluorescent colors, as the standard for its police vehicles and ambulances **FIGURE 4-2** .

Because the Battenburg pattern is not recognized in the United States, researchers looked at the chevron pattern, which is generally thought to signal danger **FIGURE 4-3** .[4] According to

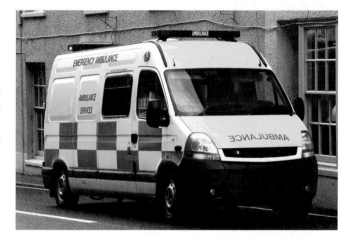

Figure 4-2 The United Kingdom has used the Battenburg pattern, alternating contrasting fluorescent colors, as the standard for its police vehicles and ambulances since 2000.

© TACrafts/iStockphoto

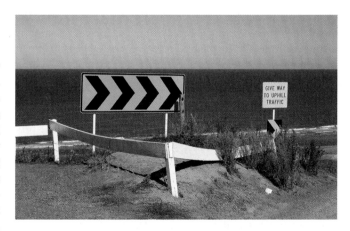

Figure 4-3 The chevron pattern indicates danger.

© meredithbarcham/iStockphoto

NFPA 1901: Standard for Automotive Fire Apparatus, fire service vehicles purchased since 2009 have been required to have at least 50% of the rear vertical surface covered with the inverted V chevron pattern. The 2013 edition of NFPA 1917: Standard for Automotive Ambulances requires ambulances to have at least the same pattern.

Retroreflective material offers another level of vehicle conspicuity. All too often, nighttime drivers have difficulty determining vehicle direction and motion. Outlining the contour edges of the emergency vehicle with retroreflective materials will improve drivers' ability to see EMS vehicles. Combining all aspects of fluorescent colors, patterns, and reflectivity should provide a greater distance of visibility to other drivers and provide greater reaction time to avoid possible collisions with EMS vehicles on roadway scenes.

Arrival and Scene Size-Up

When responding to a roadway incident, you need to plan how you will help control the scene and help provide maximum protection to the emergency responders, patients, and bystanders. You must help control the environment in which you will operate. This step is part of the scene size-up and must be accomplished before you step out of the ambulance.

If your ambulance is first on the scene, park uphill and upwind of the scene. Many agencies require parking the ambulance in front of the incident and the larger, heavier fire apparatus behind the incident, thus protecting the transporting ambulance. This also protects the EMS practitioners performing patient loading from oncoming traffic. Always follow your agency's policies and procedures.

If your ambulance responds to a scene with law enforcement and fire apparatus already present, the fire apparatus should encircle the incident scene and block it off from all roadway traffic **FIGURE 4-4** .[5] If the incident command system has been activated, check with the incident commander on where to park the ambulance. Ambulances should park at a 45-degree angle in front of the vehicles involved in the incident. The wheels of the ambulance should be angled away from the incident scene. By angling the ambulance wheels away from the incident scene, if the ambulance is hit by a distracted driver, the ambulance will be pushed out into the roadway instead of into the incident scene and potentially those working there. The doors to the patient compartment should be facing the incident scene so the ambulance crew and the patient will be protected during loading procedures. After parking the ambulance, let any EMS practitioners riding in the patient care compartment know which door to exit so they can avoid stepping into traffic.

Law enforcement should set up flares or traffic cones as line **tapering** to warn drivers that they are approaching emergency operations and should slow down and move over one lane **FIGURE 4-5** . This will help give emergency responders the room to work safely. In addition, law enforcement may

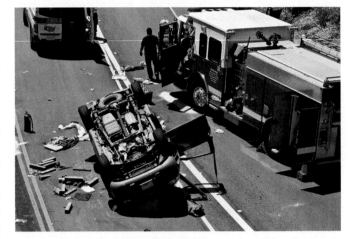

Figure 4-4 Fire apparatus should encircle the incident scene and block it off from all roadway traffic.
© pbk-pg/Shutterstock

close additional lanes, stop traffic, and even close access to sections of the road entirely. If the situation requires it, additional resources should be requested to implement traffic control measures that may include electronic signage **FIGURE 4-6** . How law enforcement responds should be spelled out in the local TIM plan.

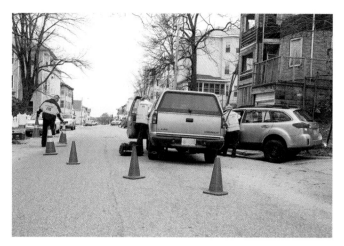

Figure 4-5 Line tapering can help protect responders from oncoming traffic.

© Jones & Bartlett Learning. Photographed by Darren Stahlman.

Before exiting the vehicle, don high-visibility safety apparel. A typical EMS uniform is dark pants, dark shirt, and dark jacket. This ensemble does not do anything to enhance the visibility of the EMS practitioner. In 2008, federal regulation 23CFR634 went into effect, mandating that anyone working in the right-of-way of a federal aid highway must wear high-visibility clothing, including vests, that meets the requirements of the American National Standards Institute (ANSI) FIGURE 4-7 . This requirement applies to all emergency responders, including EMS practitioners, whether paid or volunteer. Today, the high-visibility safety apparel worn most by EMS professionals is an ANSI-compliant safety vest because it can be worn over any garment any time of the year, versus jackets that are typically only worn in cooler temperatures.

High-visibility safety vests and clothing must be worn in the day and night. High-visibility vests have instantly recognizable fluorescent backgrounds and reflective strips. High-visibility clothing, including the turnout gear for fire fighters, includes reflective strips and trim. Most fire fighter turnout gear does not meet this requirement; therefore, the responding fire fighters should still don high-visibility apparel on top of their turnout gear.

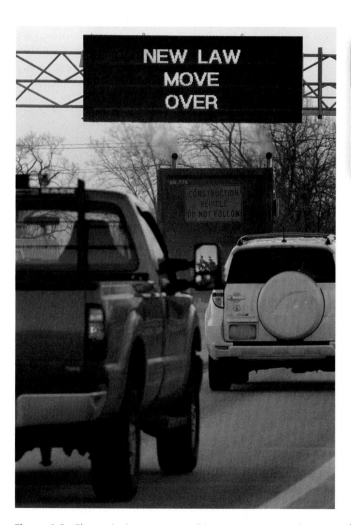

Figure 4-6 Electronic signs can warn drivers to move over a lane to give emergency responders the room to work safely.

© David Duprey/AP Photo

IN THE FIELD

Traffic control is vital to the safety of emergency responders, patients, and bystanders and should always be rendered to the local law enforcement authority.

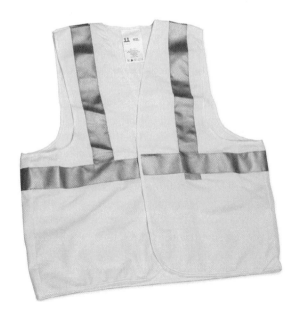

Figure 4-7 All EMS practitioners must wear high-visibility apparel when responding to roadway incidents.

© Tsuji/iStockphoto

Before stepping out of the ambulance, ensure that no traffic is coming. Just as you use your mirrors when driving to ensure that it is safe to change lanes, check your mirrors and your blind spot to see if it is safe to exit the ambulance. If your view is still unclear, crack open the door to see if the path is clear. When you exit the ambulance, remember to stay close to it and keep your eyes on the road for any traffic.

Operations

The goal of operations is to clear the scene as quickly as possible. EMS practitioners and emergency responders should never

respond to highway operations in privately owned vehicles because they typically do not have adequate warning lights and visibility profiles.

Emergency Lighting
More May Not Be Better

Different lighting modes have different purposes. In addition, the type and number of lights have varying results. Research by the National Institute of Standards and Technology has shown that as the number of flashing lights increases, the ability of drivers to quickly respond to the emergency message decreases.[6] Too much lighting can also cause emergency responders to "get lost" in the scene clutter, increasing their risk of being hit by a vehicle. Additionally, modern emergency lights are extremely bright and can cause night blindness as drivers pass by the scene, potentially causing additional incidents down the road.

On-Scene Lighting Modes

It is important to use proper lighting on the highway. When possible, clear (white) lights should not be projected toward oncoming traffic to avoid blinding drivers. This includes the headlights of emergency vehicles. Also be cognizant of the intensity of modern-day strobe lights and their effect on traffic approaching the scene from both directions.

If your ambulance is equipped with an Opticom device, it should be off. If the ambulance's Opticom is left on while parked at an intersection, it will continue to override the nearest intersection's traffic signal, causing increased traffic congestion.

Air Ambulance

The decision to use an air ambulance is determined by a number of factors, including patient status, the distance to the most appropriate facility, and protocol. If the decision to launch a helicopter is made, typically the incident commander will have his or her team set up a landing zone (LZ) near the incident, as appropriate for the surroundings and size of the incoming aircraft. Once on the ground, the EMS crew and flight crew will coordinate loading the patient into the aircraft using the flight crew litter.

Most aircraft will be on the ground "hot," or with the engine(s) on. Because of this, particular procedures must be followed when approaching the aircraft. Each aircraft is different, and the procedures will be spelled out by the air crew. Familiarize yourself with your local procedures for approaching and loading an air ambulance.

STAY IN THE FIELD

Every EMS system at some point will respond to a call on a roadway, be it an MVC, a medical case in a vehicle that has pulled over to the side of the road, or a pedestrian struck by a vehicle. Operating at the scene of these calls places emergency responders in an unprotected environment where there is great potential for additional injuries caused by distracted drivers. As EMS practitioners, we need to use every method available to protect ourselves from becoming another statistic. We can do this by embracing the tools we have, including the use of vehicle positioning, high-visibility clothing, enhanced situational awareness, interagency cooperation, and a change in our attitudes toward safety.

WRAP-UP

Summary

- EMS practitioners too often become victims themselves when distracted drivers fail to see them and strike them with their vehicles.
- Roadway operations pose significant risks to EMS practitioners and other responders, as well as to patients and bystanders.
- All emergency responders need to work together in our approach and management of roadway incidents to improve scene safety for all. This includes changing individual beliefs from "It can't happen to me" to "What can I do to prevent it from happening to me?"
- A Traffic Incident Management (TIM) plan is a pre-planning document created with the input of all emergency responding agencies. A TIM plan ensures that all agencies will work together to secure the scene, maintain scene safety, care for and safely extract patients from the scene, and clear the scene as efficiently and safely as possible.
- In 2009, the Emergency Vehicle Visibility and Conspicuity Study (FA-323) discussed the importance of enhancing vehicle visibility using conspicuity products. Enhancing a vehicle's conspicuity is not just about making it easily visible but also about enhancing the safety of the ambulance.
- When responding to a roadway incident, you need to plan how you will help control the scene and help provide maximum protection to the emergency responders, patients, and bystanders. You must help control the environment in which you will operate.
- If your ambulance is first on the scene, park uphill and upwind of the scene.
- If your ambulance responds to a scene with law enforcement and fire apparatus already present, the fire apparatus should encircle the incident scene and block it off from all roadway traffic.
- If the incident command system has been activated, check with the incident commander on where to park the ambulance.
- Ambulances should park at a 45-degree angle in front of the vehicles involved in the incident.
- The doors to the patient compartment should be facing the incident scene so that the ambulance crew and the patient will be protected during loading procedures.
- Before exiting the vehicle, don high-visibility safety apparel. High-visibility safety vests and clothing must be worn during the day and at night.
- Before stepping out of the ambulance, ensure that no traffic is coming.
- When you exit the ambulance, remember to stay close to it and keep your eyes on the road for any traffic.
- The goal of operations is to clear the scene as quickly as possible.
- Too much lighting can also cause emergency responders to "get lost" in the scene clutter, increasing their risk of being hit by a vehicle. When possible, clear (white) lights should not be projected toward oncoming traffic to avoid blinding drivers.
- If the decision to launch an air ambulance is made, typically the incident commander will have his or her team set up a landing zone near the incident. Once on the ground, the EMS crew and flight crew will coordinate loading the patient into the aircraft using the flight crew litter. Familiarize yourself with your local procedures for approaching and loading an air ambulance.

WRAP-UP (CONTINUED)

Glossary

conspicuity The ability of a vehicle to draw the attention of other drivers.

tapering A method to gradually direct traffic flow into an unaffected lane.

Traffic Incident Management (TIM) plan A preplanning document created with the input of all emergency responding agencies that ensures that all agencies will work together to secure the scene, maintain scene safety, care for and safely extract patients from the scene, and clear the scene as efficiently and safely as possible.

WRAP-UP (CONTINUED)

References

1. National Highway Traffic Safety Administration. *Traffic Safety Facts 2012: A Compilation of Motor Vehicle Crash Data from the Fatality Analysis Reporting System and the General Estimates System.* U.S. Department of Transportation. Washington, DC: National Highway Traffic Safety Administration; 2012. http://www.nrd-nhtsa.dot.gov/8102046.pdf. Accessed June 9, 2015.
2. National Highway Institute. *National Traffic Incident Management Responder Training Program: Train-the-Trainer Guide.* Washington, DC: National Highway Institute; 2013.
3. De Lorenzo R, Eilers M. Lights and sirens: a review of emergency vehicle warning systems. *Ann Emerg Med.* 1991;20(12):1331–1335.
4. Federal Emergency Management Association. Emergency Vehicle Visibility and Conspicuity Study (FA-323). Washington, DC: U.S. Department of Homeland Security; 2009.
5. State of New Jersey. New Jersey Highway Incident Traffic Safety Guidelines for Emergency Responders. State of New Jersey; 2010.
6. Flannagan MJ, Blower DF, Devonshire JM. *Effects of Warning Lamp Color and Intensity on Driver Vision.* Ann Arbor: University of Michigan Transportation Research Institute; 2008.

Additional Readings

1. U.S. Fire Administration. Emergency Vehicle Safety Initiative (Publication FA-336). Washington, DC: U.S. Fire Administration; 2014.

CHAPTER 5

Patient Handling

CHAPTER OBJECTIVES

After reading this chapter, the participant will be able to:

- Discuss the importance of practicing proper lifting and moving techniques to maintain the safety of both the patient and the EMS practitioner

- Discuss the consequences to the patient of improper lifting and moving techniques

- Discuss the risks for and the consequences of back injury for the EMS practitioner

- Discuss the best practices for lifting and moving patients

- Describe how to evaluate the patient to determine the requirements for safe movement

- Describe how to evaluate the environment for hazards that could impede the safe lifting and moving of a patient

- Describe how to develop a safe lifting and moving plan for each patient

- Discuss the possible lifting and moving equipment options that could be used in the application of a lifting and moving plan

- Discuss the maintenance of patient lifting and moving equipment

© Barbol/Shutterstock

SCENARIO

At the end of your 24-hour shift, you are dispatched to an extended care facility to transport a stretcher-bound patient to dialysis. You and your partner arrive to find the patient unresponsive. After obtaining the transfer report, you place the stack of paperwork under the patient's feet.

Your partner takes the position at the head of the stretcher, and you exit the facility with the patient. As you guide the stretcher down the bumpy sidewalk, you notice that the paperwork is flying away. Without speaking, you let go of the stretcher to chase down the paperwork. Your partner sees the paperwork out of the corner of her eye, and without speaking, she lets go of the stretcher to chase it down. The stretcher continues down the sidewalk and stops suddenly when the wheel hits a large bump. The stretcher tips over, and the patient remains attached to the stretcher. However, he bumps his head on the curb and sustains a subdural hematoma.

1. What errors were made?
2. What could have been done differently?
3. How does situational awareness apply here?

Introduction

Patient handling is a critical component in all forms of medical transportation **FIGURE 5-1**. Improper patient handling introduces an unacceptable level of risk for the patient and the EMS practitioner. It may also negate the effects of clinical interventions. For example, the rough handling of a splinted extremity will increase the patient's pain, thus negating one of the reasons that a splint is applied: to reduce the level of pain from an injury.

Even when performed properly, lifting exposes the EMS practitioner to the cumulative effects of mechanical stressors. Consequently, minimizing lifting is a goal for each patient movement event.

Hazards to patient movement, such as an icy sidewalk, must be recognized and removed. This requires a thoughtful analysis of each situation before lifting and moving the patient. Before a patient is moved, a "diagnosis" must take place in which the EMS practitioners assess the specific patient and the environmental factors to develop a "care plan" for patient movement. This chapter discusses how to perform these evaluations and create a safe and efficient plan for lifting and moving. It also covers the use of mechanical and lateral transfer aids and how to maintain lifting and moving equipment.

IN THE FIELD

Situational awareness is vital to safe stretcher operations.

STAY IN THE FIELD

Before moving the patient, you need to apply your critical thinking skills and anticipate everything that *could* happen during the move. Any potential hazards need to be eliminated before the move.

Safe Patient Movement

Safe patient movement is critical for EMS practitioners because we have an obligation to our patients to "Primum, non nocere." This is loosely translated as "At first, do no harm." The literal translation is "At first, not to kill." Improper patient movement can kill

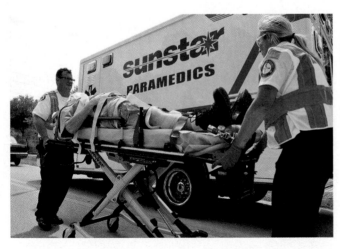

Figure 5-1 Patient handling is a critical component in all forms of medical transportation.
© Courtesy of Sunstar Paramedics.

patients. It does not take a dramatic stretcher (or cot, litter, or gurney) collapse or dropping someone down some stairs for a death to occur. Always keep in mind how fragile some of our patients are.

For example, dialysis patients receive anticoagulants to maintain the patency of their arteriovenous access lines. This makes them especially vulnerable to injury. Events that would be harmless to a patient not receiving anticoagulants can cause significant injury in a patient receiving them. For example, a low-impact "bump" on the head might cause a superficial bruise in a patient who is not receiving anticoagulants, whereas a patient receiving anticoagulants could sustain a subdural hematoma.

Safety Begins with You

As EMS practitioners, our focus on patient safety may make us give inadequate attention to our own well-being while lifting and moving a patient. Remember, even healthy bodies are at risk for injury. The spine and joints are particularly susceptible to injury from lifting. EMS practitioners are no strangers to the acute pain of sprains and strains, and not all damage to the body is accompanied by acute pain. Even if you lift patients perfectly throughout your career, the cumulative effects of lifting and moving heavy loads can lead to injury **FIGURE 5-2**. To prevent both the cumulative effects and immediate, catastrophic effects, minimize both the load and the number of times that you lift.

Unsafe Patient Handling: Physical and Psychological Harm to Patients

In addition to physical injury, unsafe patient handling may cause discomfort. Vertical and lateral stretcher drops, bumpy rides, rapid elevation changes, and detachment from the stretcher may frighten patients. The natural autonomic nervous system sympathetic response may raise the heart rate and blood pressure for both the patient and EMS practitioner. Is it reasonable to raise the myocardial oxygen consumption of a patient during a routine transfer? How will the additional stress impact you? Your patient may become less cooperative, making your job more challenging. In addition, the strain of the patient's autonomic nervous system sympathetic response may worsen the patient's condition.

Pediatric Patients

Pediatric patients are a challenge. In most patient populations, they are a distinct minority. Psychomotor skills with pediatric patients require constant practice. Some EMS practitioners may not be entirely comfortable with pediatric-specific equipment because they have limited experience with it. Now imagine a child trying to process all the novel information that comes with an ambulance ride **FIGURE 5-3**. If a child is frightened by an improper movement, will he or she be very likely to cooperate during clinical interventions?

Bariatric Patients

Bariatric patients are more prevalent than ever. About 1 adult man in 80 weighs over 300 pounds, while 1 adult woman in 200 is 300 pounds or heavier. Part of caring for bariatric patients is protecting their dignity and treating them in a nonjudgmental fashion. In a society that aggressively values thinness, people who are in the opposite weight extreme may have psychological issues with self-esteem. Any errors in movement may be more difficult to correct and may cause injury to the patient and the EMS practitioner.

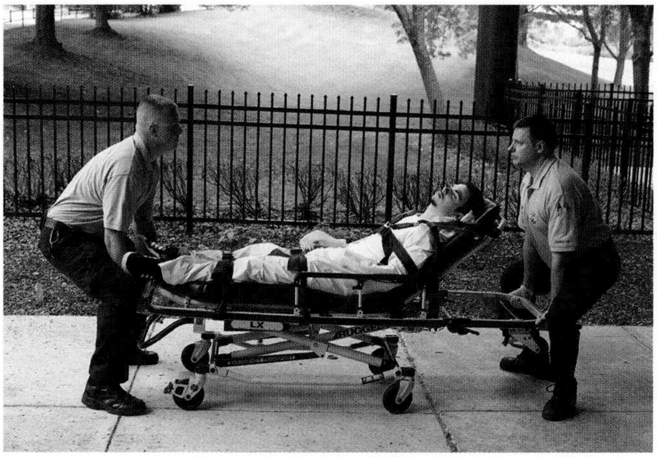

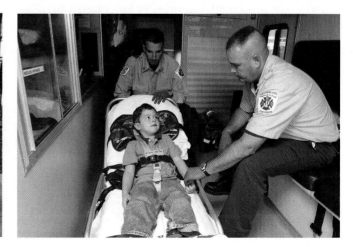

Figure 5-2 Even if your body is perfectly aligned during each and every lift, the cumulative effects of lifting and moving heavy loads can lead to injury.

© Jones & Bartlett Learning.

Figure 5-3 Pediatric patients may be as uncomfortable riding in an ambulance as some EMS practitioners are with pediatric-specific equipment.

© Jones & Bartlett Learning.

Geriatric Patients

Geriatric patients may be impaired in the way that they process environmental cues. Vision, hearing, balance, and, in some cases, proprioception, or sense of orientation, deteriorate with age. This awkwardness creates an enhanced sensitivity to movement. Because they may not be able to adequately process what they see, hear, or feel, geriatric patients may not be able to communicate their source of discomfort. It is not uncommon for geriatric patients to feel that they are losing control. Any clumsiness that we exhibit during routine movements will diminish their confidence in us, impair our ability to control the situation, and lessen the likelihood that we can implement safe lifting practices efficiently.

Unsafe Patient Handling: Physical and Psychological Harm to EMS Practitioners
The Risks and Consequences of Back Injury

According to a 2007 article in the *American Journal of Industrial Medicine*, about 10% of the EMS workforce is out at any given time because of illness or injury.[1] Unfortunately, this number is currently cited as accurate.

There is an apparent epidemic of back injuries in EMS. Consider the following:

- Back injury is the top reason for seeing a doctor.[2]
- Back injury is the most common cause of disability.[3]
- Half of all EMS practitioners are affected by some degree of back injury.[4]
- Back injury is the top reason for leaving EMS.[5]
- Back injury is often the result of cumulative wear and tear.

The occurrence of back injury has been related to high call volume, which in this context was defined as 40 or more calls per week. EMS workers in communities with a population of 25,000 or more were 3 times more likely to report an injury than those in a rural environment.[1]

Many critical risk factors contribute to back injury. Uncoordinated lifts due to height disparities, fatigue, injured team members, or poor communication may cause uneven distribution of the load, causing those lifting to strain or move into awkward positions. Personnel may be exposed to environmental hazards such as slick, uneven, or rough surfaces. The intervention of those untrained in safe lifting techniques may alter the load distribution and interfere with the proper use of equipment. Explicit instructions should be given to everyone who will be assisting in the lift.

STAY IN THE FIELD

Many fitness programs can make you stronger. Bryan Fass, who developed the Fit Responder Course, adds that weak abdominal, pelvic, hip, and gluteal muscles lack the endurance to do their job throughout the day, so they place an extra load on the muscles of the spine and back. Keeping your core strong is important in protecting your back.

You should exercise to increase your endurance, but strength alone will not keep you injury free. You need to have the strength to do your job, but you also need the flexibility. To keep your muscles active, functioning, and ready to lift, it is vital to stretch at the beginning of your shift and several times throughout. Flexibility and mobility increase with stretching and elongating the muscles that shorten when they are not being used. Feet, ankles, hamstrings, hip flexors, and pectoral and gluteal muscles are our workhorses. We would not expect to run a marathon without proper stretching and maintenance, yet we expect our bodies to be in peak performance in our job without taking care of them. Quite often we take better care of our vehicles than we do our bodies, and we expect our bodies to last throughout our careers.

STAY IN THE FIELD

Lumbar spine, shoulder, and knee injuries may range from simple strains or sprains to major anatomic injury, such as tears, disruptions of joint spaces, and fractures. In addition, remember that lifting can have cumulative effects that result in back pathologies even when performed correctly.

Finally, remember that a warm muscle is 25% more effective than a cold muscle. Simple foot, ankle, hamstring, hip, and gluteal stretches will help to prevent injuries.

The Direct and Indirect Costs of Back Injury

Direct costs are those commonly associated with out-of-pocket payments. They include payments to physicians, rehabilitation professionals, insurance carriers, and attorneys. Other direct costs are compensatory salaries for lost work and employee replacement costs. The financial impact to an EMS practitioner can be devastating.

In terms of actual dollars, it is estimated that a simple lumbar sprain will have an average direct cost of $18,365.[6] A more complicated back injury can have direct costs of $100,000 per year.[7] Subsequent back injuries can cost the system 2 to 4 times the initial injury.[2]

One way to look at direct costs is to think of them as what it takes to make the physical pain and disability go away. It seems that it would be smarter to avoid the pain and disability, skip the suffering, and save the money through utilizing preventive techniques that minimize lifting, such as lift assist teams and patient-handling equipment and devices.

Indirect costs may be 15 to 40 times greater than direct costs.[3] Indirect costs are those expenses that society incurs when you have a debilitating injury that does not allow you to be you. Your inability to function at home costs money and creates psychological pain for your family. How does your injury alter the way your significant other and children live? What adaptations do they have to make? Nobody in EMS gets rich. How many EMS practitioners work multiple jobs or take as much overtime as possible just to make ends meet? What happens if your household must manage solely on disability income, which is usually around two-thirds of base pay?

Patient Handling

Patient handling is a complex psychomotor skill that requires significant cognitive and behavioral preparation. The 2012

injury and illness data for EMS workers reveal that sprains and strains were the most common diagnosis. Most of the injuries involved bodily reactions and exertion.[9] About half of the overexertion events occurred during lifting. Surprisingly, a study in the *Journal of Occupational Medicine* showed that classes in body mechanics and training in lifting techniques improve skills in the short term but alone do not reduce injuries.[10] Follow-up studies show that emphasizing the use of task-specific patient-handling equipment, such as power-cots, antifriction devices, and bariatric devices, is mandatory, along with body mechanics training, for achieving a successful injury prevention program. The proper use of lifting and moving equipment requires training and retraining for EMS practitioners.

While we cannot completely eliminate lifting, we can identify lifting situations with higher risks and use task-specific patient-handling equipment with proper body mechanics to minimize the cumulative and acute effects of lifting—for example, using a stair chair rather than carrying a patient down stairs **FIGURE 5-4**.

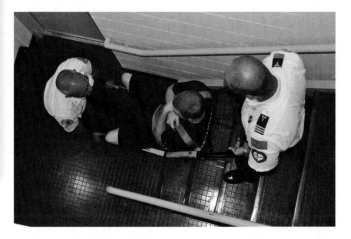

Figure 5-4 Using equipment such as a stair chair properly can help protect your back.
© Courtesy of Sunstar Paramedics.

Also, we cannot hold the misconception that injuries occur only with strenuous lifting. Injuries can occur during "routine" lifting, such as moving a 90-pound nursing home patient from a bed to a stretcher. We must use situational awareness and treat each lifting event as a potential source of injury.

Safe patient movement combines evidence-based practices, training, body maintenance, and common sense. It has been shown that formal patient lifting classes in body mechanics and training in safe lifting techniques do not reduce caregiver injuries by themselves.[10] Training is important, but it must be combined with evidence-based practices to be effective. Evidence-based practices include:

- Minimizing manual patient handling
- Utilizing lift assist/lift teams
- Employing patient and environment assessment strategies
- Utilizing patient-handling equipment and devices
- Training and retraining on lifting and equipment use
- Behavior modification
- Maintaining a healthy body, flexibility, and mobility

Minimizing Manual Patient Handling

EMS practitioner injuries from patient handling can be minimized by reducing the number of times patients are lifted and decreasing the amount of load per practitioner per lift. Patients should be allowed to help move themselves when an appropriate physical evaluation shows that it is safe to do so.

Independent of patient size, an even distribution of the load among EMS practitioners is mandatory to prevent injury. EMS practitioners have a tendency to be acutely aware of lifting only when the patient is extremely obese. Injuries are sustained when the same level of focused intensity is not given to lifting and moving smaller patients.

Utilizing Lift Assist/Lift Teams

Lift assist teams are used to supply adequate people power in the case of a heavy patient or other situations in which help is needed to safely move a patient. Lift assist teams can be made up of additional responders on the scene, hospital staff, or another ambulance crew called in as backup. The key to a successful lift assist team is practicing good communication. Everyone on the team must understand the lifting and moving plan, his or her role in the plan, and exactly when to begin lifting ("Ready, set, lift").

In addition to weight, factors such as a long distance to move the patient from the scene to the ambulance, the presence of ice or snow, and terrain issues such as hills, steps, and other inclines, require assistance. Weight should not be the *only* factor in determining the need for a lift assist.

Finally, EMS practitioners who request a lift assist should not be subjected to ridicule or denied help.

Employing Patient and Environment Assessment Strategies

As a matter of routine, we determine scene safety. We then do a quick clinical evaluation of the patient and act accordingly. Before we move the patient, we must do an assessment to determine what patient characteristics exist that direct the manner in which we can safely move him or her. Before movement, we must assess the environment to create a plan that mitigates any hazards. It is imperative to address hazards before we move the patient.

Utilizing Patient-Handling Equipment and Devices

The use of any patient-handling equipment or device must be part of a systematic approach to patient movement. The addition of devices must never create practices in which proper body mechanics are ignored. For example, powercots can weigh 60 to 80 pounds more than a regular stretcher. How do you decide whether to take the powercot to the patient, or the patient to the device?

Training and Retraining on Lifting and Equipment Use

EMS practitioners must be trained specifically on proper lifting techniques, behavior modifications, maintaining a healthy body, and techniques on maintaining mobility and flexibility as part of orientation, and they should receive refresher training at least annually. EMS practitioners should be observed during actual patient encounters, be evaluated, and receive coaching as necessary. Training and maintenance on devices should be done in

EMS agencies should develop a stretcher obstacle course with different surfaces and scenarios for use during orientation. New employees will use their critical thinking skills to determine how to safely move patients over different surfaces and during challenging scenarios **FIGURE 5-5**.

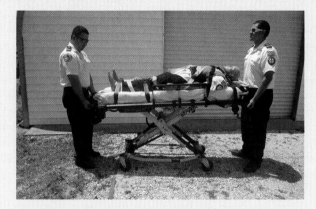

Figure 5-5 EMS agencies should develop a stretcher obstacle course with different surfaces (such as gravel) and scenarios as part of orientation.

Courtesy of Sunstar Paramedics.

When moving a patient, do not forget to use proper body mechanics each and every time. Proper body mechanics should be a habit so that when something goes wrong, your muscle memory kicks in and maintains the best form and technique. Proper body mechanics include:

- Keeping your head up and shoulders back
- Keeping your eyes on your partner's face
- Maintaining abdominal bracing (stiffening your core to apply pressure on your spine)
- Keeping your feet rooted to the floor, slightly wider than shoulder width, and toes pointed slightly outward
- Keeping your hips hinged and not pushed forward, so you can do a proper squat
- Keeping your palms faceup
- Keeping the load close to your body

Evaluation of the Patient and Environment

Patient Assessment

What do we need to know about the patient before we can move him or her safely **FIGURE 5-6**? In addition to our condition-specific clinical assessment, consider the following:

- Age (spectrum from infant to elderly)
- Ability of the patient to provide assistance (independent, partial, or dependent)
- Ability to bear weight (full, partial, or none)
- Upper extremity strength (bilateral)
- Ability and *willingness* to cooperate and follow instructions (acute chronic cognitive impairment, language barrier, or psychiatric/personality disorder)
- Height and weight (body mass index, bariatric, or cachectic [possessing an appearance of wasting away])
- Conditions likely to affect patient handling, including:
  - Amputations, spasms, fractures, joint replacement, paralysis, cardio-respiratory compromise, edema, osteoporosis, pain, urinary or fecal catheter, and very fragile skin

In other words, how does our patient assessment inform our situational awareness? Are there complicating factors? Is a patient who is usually at risk for falls more difficult to move safely? Studies have shown that people over the age of 65, with

accordance with the manufacturer's guidelines that are spelled out in the user's manual.

Behavioral Controls

Safe patient movement requires the selection of **safe patient movement behaviors**. Safe patient movement behaviors are those actions selected by the EMS practitioner that minimize the risk of injury to patients, practitioners, and bystanders during patient movement events. They include the proper evaluation of the patient and environment, acquisition of adequate resources (properly trained personnel and appropriate equipment), the use of proper body mechanics, and ongoing communication among team members and the patient. This is achieved in part through the implementation of behavioral controls.

Behavioral controls require management, oversight, enforcement, and example to create a culture of safety. Patient and environmental assessments are examples of behavioral controls. Education and training are not effective if the desired behaviors do not exist. EMS practitioners should take pride and ownership in how a patient is handled and treated.

Safe patient movement behaviors can only be performed by EMS practitioners who know what to do, are physically capable of doing it, and, most important, want to do it safely.

multiple diagnoses, a history of falls over the past 3 months, incontinence, vision impairment, impaired functional mobility, polypharmacy (four or more prescriptions), postural hypotension, and fear of falling are at increased risk of falling.

Safe patient movement is also impacted by special circumstances that are likely to affect transfer or repositioning tasks, such as wounds, tubes, and other medical equipment, attached or implanted. Physician orders or recommendations of ancillary personnel regarding transferring or repositioning patients may be needed in the context of recent joint replacement or fractures. Specific angles of extension or abduction are sometimes used to maintain orthopedic integrity.

After determining our patient's needs, we must evaluate the environment.

Environmental Assessment

We must perform the environmental assessment to determine how the environment will impact safe patient movement FIGURE 5-7 :

- Presence of fixed physical obstructions (things we cannot move)
- Presence of removable physical obstructions
- Terrain that requires lifting and carrying the patient to the transport medium (e.g., stretcher, stair chair)
- Terrain that makes the use of good body mechanics difficult
- Distance the patient must be lifted or carried
- Adequate lighting
- Freedom from bystander interference
- Factors that limit the use of **engineering controls**, or changes made to the work environment through the use of equipment to avoid work-related injury (e.g., specialty stretchers, lateral transfer aids)

Have you ever had a patient on a stretcher and, while trying to get the patient to the ambulance, found your path blocked? There are two kinds of obstructions to consider. Fixed physical obstructions are those that we cannot move. Discovering a fixed obstruction requires us to plan how to get around it. Movable physical obstructions are those that can be removed from our path. Isn't it a good idea to move objects *before* we reach them with a patient on a stretcher?

Is there terrain that requires lifting and carrying the patient to the transport medium? When do we take the stretcher to the patient, or the patient to the stretcher? A stretcher should never be taken up a flight of stairs (or five risers). Think about what is physically easier. If stairs are involved, the added weight of the powercot may make a stair chair a better choice. How far must the patient be lifted or carried? Does the terrain make the use of good body mechanics difficult? A steep or slanted incline, a rough or slick surface, or cramped quarters may make it difficult to get into a proper lifting position. Think of building terrain, not just the outdoors. Is the lighting adequate? Are we free from bystander interference? Are there factors that limit our ability to use equipment? Narrow hallways and small rooms may require us to move the patient to the equipment.

Once we obtain the information from our assessments of the patient and the environment, we are ready to process the information and act on it. We do so by forming a plan.

STAY IN THE FIELD

Using equipment such as a Reeves cot or patient mover mat can help you when moving a patient in tight quarters.

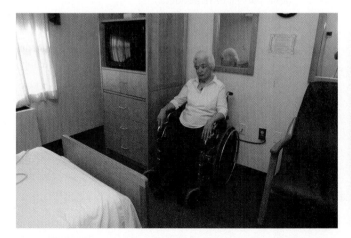

Figure 5-6 What do you need to know about this patient before you can move her safely?

© Jones & Bartlett Learning.

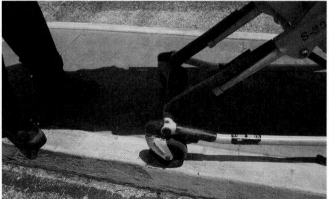

Figure 5-7 What are the potential hazards in this environment?

© Courtesy of Sunstar Paramedics.

Form a Lifting and Moving Plan

To form a lifting and moving plan, we must ask ourselves four questions.

1. As a result of our environmental assessment, what do we need to address before we move the patient?
2. Based on the patient assessment, what do we need to address before we move the patient?
3. Can personnel on the scene safely lift the patient and the necessary equipment without overexerting themselves?
4. What task-specific equipment and personnel will be required to safely move the patient in each phase of the event: transfer, securement, transport, loading, and unloading?

STAY IN THE FIELD

Lifting from below the knees, which is inherently dangerous, exposes the spine and lower back to extreme compressive loads that exceed both the Federal Emergency Management Agency (FEMA) and NIOSH recommendations for safe lifting. Using devices like flexible stretchers, lift extenders, and other approved devices will drastically reduce your exposure to injurious loads by allowing you to lift a patient as a team with your hands at roughly knee height instead of off the floor.

Question 1: Environment

What is our initial impression? Are there weather or hazardous materials issues? Is a police or fire presence needed? Have we adequately assessed the terrain and distance? Have we removed obstacles, planned our route, and selected the proper equipment? Naturally, the site needs to be safe before we enter it, but we must also be able to leave the scene safely. Using the information gathered in the environmental assessment, we will communicate with our team members, request their feedback, and then collectively form a plan of action. Communication is key throughout the process.

Any request for police, fire, or additional manpower will be made. We will note the conditions of the area between our unit and the patient. Before moving the patient, we will remove anything we can that obstructs our access. A plan for going around fixed obstructions will be made—for example, "We'll stay on the lower side of the boulder."

Any slick, rough, or uneven areas will be noted and communicated among the team. Constant scene size-up is required. While a scene may initially be free from bystander interference, the arrival of bystanders may require police intervention. A decision will be made about how equipment will be used. "We'll sit him upright in the bed and rotate him onto a stair chair. We'll take him down the stairs on the stair chair and put him on the stretcher in the living room. The porch light is out, so we'll have his daughter shine the flashlight on the steps."

Question 2: Patient

Is there a need for immediate patient removal because of hazards, toxins, fire, hostile bystanders, or other dangers? Is there a clinical indication for "load and go," or do we need to stabilize the patient medically before transport?

Do we need to discuss with the patient, family, or other EMS practitioners the effects of any cognitive, communicative, or physical impairments the patient may be exhibiting? Are there medical equipment issues? Are there any clinical conditions that require special positions? Have we considered language barriers or any special needs?

Conditions that take precedence over patient movement issues include dangerous scenes and critical clinical conditions that require immediate transport. Situational awareness and common sense allow us to recognize physical threats. Protocols and communication with medical control help with the clinical concerns.

We must establish effective communication with our patient. If dementia or other forms of cognitive impairment make the patient unable to follow directions, precautions such as the use of restraints or the presence of a caretaker may be needed. Do we have a rudimentary understanding of the languages spoken by our patient population? If not, do we have immediate access to an interpreter?

Are there physical impairments that require special positioning? Think about amputation, spasms, fractures, joint replacement, paralysis, cardiorespiratory compromise, edema, osteoporosis, pain, urinary or fecal catheter, and very fragile skin.

Question 3: Personnel Preparation

The number of personnel needed should be determined *before* the lift is attempted. Perform a test lift to see if the team can safely handle the load of the patient or if backup lifters are needed. Consider the size of the patient and the previously mentioned patient and environmental characteristics.

Decide how many people will be needed in each phase. For example, how many people can initially make physical contact with the patient? What devices will be used to move the patient? If we are going down stairs, how many people will the staircase accommodate? In addition to the people actually moving the patient, how much backup do we need to provide physical support and guidance?

Share the Load

In those circumstances that require lifting, a good principle is to **share the load** by using an adequate number of personnel. The goal of the use of a lift assistor or lift assist team is to eliminate critical risk factors that contribute to back injury, including cumulative effects FIGURE 5-8 .

The risk of uncoordinated lifts by unprotected personnel is straightforward. Disparities occur when there is a size or strength mismatch between partners or among team members that is not taken into consideration before executing the lifting process. Team members who are injured or fatigued and do not share that information make it impossible to safely share the load.

Untrained or nonprofessional lifters should be avoided, but when circumstances mandate their use, they should be given specific instructions, and the team leader should make certain that the instructions are understood.

Poor communication among EMS professionals can be dangerous for the EMS practitioners and the patient. The first time a team lifts a stretcher, a patient should not be on it. At the beginning of the shift and as part of the inspection process, the ambulance crew should unload and load the stretcher. They should talk about how they will communicate, and describe their preferences and weaknesses. For example, "We'll lift on 'Lift' and always make eye contact when communicating." Poor communication results in poor execution. Ambulance crews should engage in regular practice with equipment that is not used frequently.

The physical condition of the team members, an understanding of the limitations of the physical compatibility of the lifting team, and good communication are mandatory so that all lifters perform the following tasks simultaneously:

- Maintain balance
- Heads up and eyes looking at the partner's face
- Team members in position and acknowledging that they are ready to lift

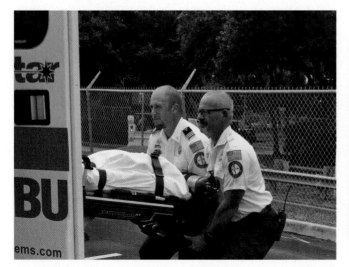

Figure 5-8 To prevent injury to the patient or personnel, always share the load.

© Courtesy of Sunstar Paramedics.

- All hands on the lifting equipment before the lift
- Use the power grip with the palms up FIGURE 5-9
- Keep the feet apart and staggered at shoulder width apart FIGURE 5-10

STAY IN THE FIELD

Too often, EMS practitioners will rush their lifts and transfers because they hold the erroneous idea that speed will make the movement easier. In many cases, slowing down and breaking up the patient lifts into two steps will make the lift safer and reduce the strain on the spine and extremity joints.

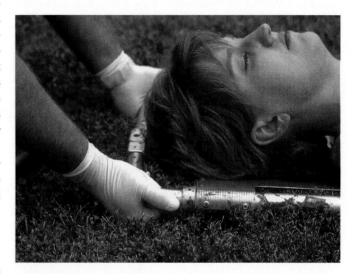

Figure 5-9 Use the power grip with your palms up when lifting.

© Jones & Bartlett Learning. Courtesy of MIEMSS.

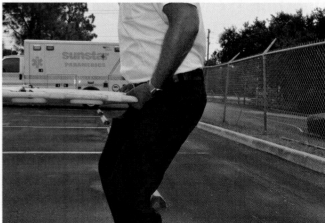

Figure 5-10 To protect your back, bend at the knees, and keep your feet apart and staggered shoulder width apart.

© Courtesy of Sunstar Paramedics.

- Do not twist
- Bend at the knees
- Maintain the lumbar curve with the torso upright
- Hold the load close to the body
- Do a small test lift, lifting the load up and down a few inches to ensure that the team can handle the weight
- Rise slowly

Body Positioning

Body positioning is as critical as sharing the load. If you are using a manual stretcher, lifts should be performed in steps to account for the changes in your body position. You should not lift the manual stretcher from the ground to the load position in one move. The movement should be to lift from the ground to the knees, stop, reposition, and then lift from the knees to the hips.

Before lifting the patient or transferring the patient vertically, position your body correctly. Assume a wide base of support with your heels down. Your hips must be hinged, your knees bent and in a mini-squat, and your chest up at all times. The biggest error that EMS practitioners make is to "look down and round" during patient lifts and transfers. Always attempt to look up or straight ahead and keep your chest up.

When moving a patient who is stabilized on a backboard laterally from one surface to another, slightly turn your foot to the direction you will be moving to eliminate twisting.

Question 4: Equipment

Equipment selection should be part of an overall patient movement plan. There are many devices used in EMS for lifting and moving patients. The pool of equipment is constantly evolving. Not all equipment will be available, or appropriate, for everyone. The selection of equipment should be based on the environment in which you work and your patient population, workforce, and availability of funds. The safety of patients and personnel

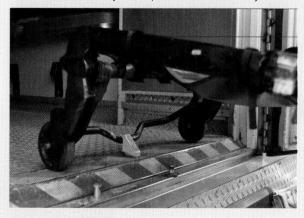

determines which equipment is purchased and how it is used. Examples of lifting and moving equipment are:

- Extrication vests, long and short spine boards, Reeves cots, patient mover tarps, scoop baskets, pole stretchers, and specialty extrication devices are used when anatomic alignment must be maintained to avoid further injury FIGURE 5-12. The use of these devices is a matter of ongoing discussion throughout the EMS community.
- Tracked and standard stair chairs and manual or powered chair cots are used to facilitate transport from the site where a patient is discovered to a secondary mode of transport FIGURE 5-13. These options are used when the stretcher is too large to place proximate to the patient or it is safer to transport the patient down stairs or rough terrain.
- Friction-reducing devices, commonly referred to as lateral transfer aids, are used to make it more comfortable for the patient and safer for the EMS practitioner when moving the patient from a surface to a stretcher. Examples of friction-reducing devices are transfer sheets, transfer boards, inflatable devices that float the patient, and mechanical lateral assist devices FIGURE 5-14.
- Ambulance stretchers may have many differences. Familiarize yourself with the operational characteristics of each.
- A variety of powered stretchers that minimize lifting are available FIGURE 5-15. They have the potential to make

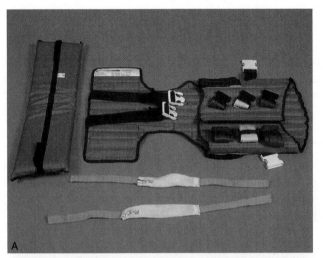
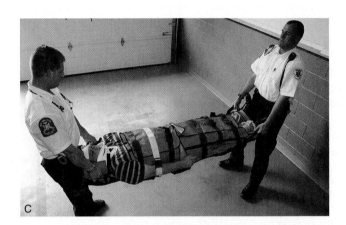
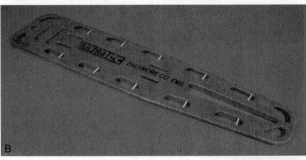
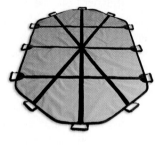

Figure 5-12 A. A vest-type immobilization device. B. A long spine board. C. A Reeves cot. D. A patient mover tarp. E. A scoop stretcher.

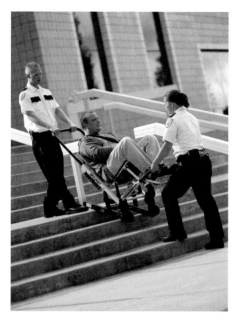

Figure 5-13 Stair chair.

Courtesy of Stryker EMS.

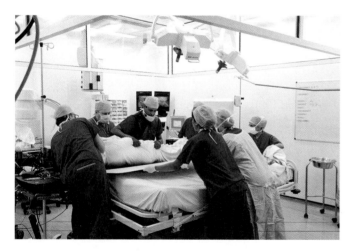

Figure 5-14 A transfer board.

© Mark Thomas/Science Source.

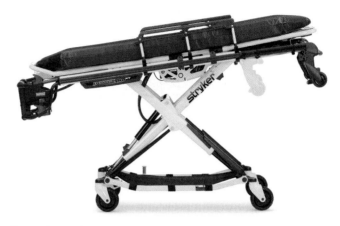

Figure 5-15 A powercot.

© Courtesy of Stryker Medical

height transitions easier for the patient. Powercots have a variety of weight capacities. Those structured for heavy loads—300 to 800 pounds—are designed to minimize lifting and are called bariatric stretchers. Bariatric stretchers are designed for bariatric patients **FIGURE 5-16**. Some bariatric patients and the equipment best suited for them will not fit in a standard ambulance; there are bariatric vehicles that meet the space requirements. Some vehicles have ramps to facilitate loading, and others have ramps with winches.

- Pediatric patients require specially designed restraint systems. Equipment designed for adults should not be used on children. Furthermore, equipment designed for and sized for pediatric patients is essential for each EMS agency. Pediatric patients should never be transported on the lap of a parent or caregiver. Pediatric patients must be secured on the stretcher in a pediatric-specific device or seat to keep them safe in the event of a collision. The selection of equipment for pediatric patients should be made under the guidance of local

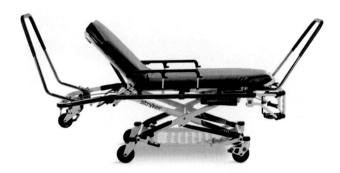

Figure 5-16 A bariatric stretcher.

© Courtesy of Stryker Medical.

medical control. Training on the use of such devices should be done by properly certified personnel.

- Stretcher retention systems should be maintained according to manufacturers' guidelines. The system selected must be compatible with the stretchers attached to them. They should be inspected by properly trained personnel routinely and after any collision.

Equipment Maintenance

EMS practitioners have the responsibility to deal with equipment within the limits of their training. This is particularly important with cleaning and maintenance. The increasing complexity of lifting and moving devices requires specialized training to safely maintain and repair them. The EMS practitioner must be familiar with the normal functionality of all equipment and immediately report any concerns. Out-of-service equipment should be clearly identified so it is not used until it is repaired.

IN THE FIELD

The useful life and the length of time it is safe to use a product should be noted at the time of purchase when applicable, and tracked.

WRAP-UP

Summary

- Safe patient movement is critical for EMS practitioners because improper patient movement can kill patients.
- To prevent both the cumulative effects and immediate, catastrophic effects of lifting, EMS practitioners should minimize both the load and the number of times that we lift.
- In addition to physical injury, unsafe patient handling may cause discomfort and worsen the patient's condition.
- Back injuries have reached epidemic levels in EMS. Back injuries generate both direct and indirect costs to the injured EMS practitioner.
- Although lifting patients cannot be completely avoided, EMS practitioners can identify lifting situations with higher risks and use task-specific patient-handling equipment with proper body mechanics to minimize the effects of lifting on the body.
- Because injuries can occur during routine lifts, EMS practitioners must practice situational awareness and approach each lift as a potential source of injury.
- Safe patient movement combines evidence-based practices and common sense. Evidence-based practices include:
  - Minimizing manual patient handling
  - Utilizing lift assist/lift teams
  - Employing patient and environment assessment strategies
  - Utilizing patient-handling equipment and devices
  - Training and retraining on techniques and equipment use
- Before lifting a patient, EMS practitioners should evaluate both the patient and environment to determine how the patient's condition and the environment will impact the ability of the EMS practitioners to move the patient safely.
- To form a lifting and moving plan, EMS practitioners must ask four questions.
  - As a result of the environmental assessment, what needs to be addressed before moving the patient?
  - Based on the patient assessment, what needs to be addressed before moving the patient?
  - Can personnel on the scene safely lift the patient and the necessary equipment without overexerting themselves?
  - What task-specific equipment and personnel will be required to safely move the patient in each phase of the event: transfer, securement, transport, loading, and unloading?
- The EMS practitioner must be familiar with the normal functionality of all equipment and immediately report any concerns.

Glossary

cachectic Possessing an appearance of wasting away; usually associated with poor nutrition or disease.

direct costs Payments made to physicians, rehabilitation professionals, insurance carriers, and attorneys; compensatory salaries for lost work; and employee replacement costs.

engineering controls Changes made to the work environment through the use of equipment to avoid work-related injury.

indirect costs The expenses and psychosocial effects related to the loss of functionality after injury, such as the inability to function normally at home, loss of ability to perform community services, and spousal/significant other adaptation to injury.

proprioception The reception and processing of sensory information that allows an individual to have an awareness of body position.

safe patient movement behaviors Those actions selected by the EMS practitioner that minimize the risk of injury to patients, practitioners, and bystanders during patient movement events.

WRAP-UP (CONTINUED)

References

1. Studnek JR, Ferketich A, Crawford J. On the job illness and injury resulting in lost work time among a national cohort of Emergency Medical Service professionals. *Am J Ind Med.* 2007;50(12):921–931.

2. Willis MT. Compensation worsens back pain. ABCNews .com. December 4, 2001. http://abcnews.go.com/Health/Pain Management/story?id=117092&page=1. Accessed June 8, 2015.

3. Spine-health. Ergonomics of the office and workplace: an overview. http://www.spine-health.com/topics/cd/ergo/ergo01.html. Accessed June 8, 2015.

4. Sternbach RA. Survey of pain in the United States: Nuprin pain report. *Clin J Pain.* 1986;2(1):49–53.

5. National Association of Emergency Medical Technicians. EMS fitness. https://www.naemt.org/emshealthsafety/EMSFitness.aspx. Accessed June 8, 2015.

6. Fass B. Medics are not disposable: injury prevention strategies. *Fit Responder.* 2009. PowerPoint presentation.

7. Austin City Council. Employee safety. *EMS Audit.* 2001;4:50–51.

8. Oregon OSHA. Firefighter and emergency medical services ergonomics curriculum. 2008. Oregon OSHA Consultative Services. http://www.cbs.state.or.us/osha/grants/ff_ergo/index .html. Accessed June 8, 2015.

9. Centers for Disease Control and Prevention. Workplace safety & health topics: emergency medical services workers: injury and illness data: 2012. http://www.cdc.gov/niosh/topics/ems/data2012.html. Accessed June 8, 2015.

10. Feldstein A, Valanis B, Vollmer W, Stevens N, Overton C. The back injury and prevention project pilot study: assessing the effectiveness of back attack. An injury prevention program among nurses, aides, and orderlies. *J Occup Med.* 1993;35:114–120.

11. de Castro AB. Handle with care: the American Nurses Association's campaign to address work-related musculoskeletal disorders. *Online J Issues Nurs.* 2004; 25(6):357.

CHAPTER 6

Patient, Practitioner, and Bystander Safety

CHAPTER OBJECTIVES

After reading this chapter, the participant will be able to:

- Describe the precautions to take at crime scenes, including scenes with an active shooter
- Describe the precautions to follow when responding to potentially secure facilities
- Describe the communication techniques to employ to de-escalate a stressful or potentially violent patient encounter
- Describe how to identify potential attackers from patients
- Recognize the issue of violence against EMS practitioners in the field

- Define and describe excited delirium syndrome
- Describe the general guidelines on patient restraint
- Describe how to mitigate errors in patient care
- Recognize the potential for EMS practitioners to come into contact with patients with new and drug-resistant organisms
- Describe how to maintain EMS practitioner safety when coming into contact with patients with new and drug-resistant organisms

© Barbol/Shutterstock

SCENARIO

At approximately 7:00 p.m., you and your partner respond to a report of a male in his 30s who is not breathing and has a weak pulse. On arrival, the patient's mother and a friend tell you they believe it's a possible overdose. You begin basic life support (BLS) maneuvers as your partner prepares and administers Narcan. The patient begins to breathe on his own and eventually wakes on his own.

Immediately on waking, the person becomes irate and refuses further treatment. He stands, pushes you, and begins to verbally threaten you. You say, "At least let me bandage you up."

He responds with, "You touch me and I'll knock you out!" as he raises his clenched fists. He then yells, "Get out of my house!"

1. Is this person still your patient?
2. Should you follow his orders to get out of his house?
3. Should you contact law enforcement and pursue criminal charges against this patient?

Introduction

Every emergency scene has the potential to create an unsafe environment for EMS practitioners. This is why the scene size-up is the first step of the patient assessment process. Some scenes may appear safe at first but then may escalate into an unsafe situation with few or subtle warning signs. Because of this, EMS practitioners must remember that scene size-up is a dynamic, evolving practice; never take anything for granted.

Every day across the country, EMS practitioners find themselves presented with potentially violent encounters with patients they were dispatched to assist. These encounters place EMS practitioners, the patient, and even bystanders at risk. In a matter of seconds, EMS practitioners must decide if they should treat the individual as a patient in need of assistance or as an aggressive attacker. EMS practitioners must decide if they will flee the encounter or if they will stay and attempt to manage the patient. Managing this type of patient involves good communication skills and sometimes the need for physical restraints. When managing these situations, safety for everyone involved—including the patient—remains the highest priority.

Illegal substances and a push toward increased outpatient management of patients with psychiatric issues have exposed EMS practitioners to a syndrome called agitated or excited delirium. A coordinated effort between law enforcement and EMS is required to handle a patient with excited delirium. Restraint of the patient is not always the answer, but in some cases, it may be the only answer. Later in this chapter, we discuss restraint concerns and techniques.

Another aspect of safety is preventing errors during patient care. Examples of patient care errors include medication errors, treatment delays, and equipment failures. Today's EMS agencies must strive to design systems that limit the potential for such errors and provide for the safe care and transportation of their patients.

Personal Safety

The main goal of every EMS practitioner should be to go home uninjured at the end of his or her shift. Unfortunately, heroes are forgotten by most, but for a hero's family, the suffering does not end. Safety should be a lifestyle and begins as soon as you commit yourself to a career in EMS. EMS practitioners should stay abreast of emerging trends by attending continuing education programs offered by the National Association of Emergency Medical Technicians (NAEMT), attending seminars and lectures at conferences, reading journals, and talking with colleagues across the country.

In the field, EMS practitioners should develop a sense of their surroundings to recognize and anticipate possible dangers. This sense of surroundings is often referred to as situational awareness. Situational awareness allows EMS practitioners to take in information, analyze the situation, and take appropriate actions.

At the onset of the response, consider the dispatch information, plan a safe response route, and follow local traffic laws. Incidents involving law enforcement are often triggers for the heart rate to increase and the right foot to press down to the floor, but remember that speed kills. On arrival at a scene, be sure to stage the ambulance in a safe location, do not block any other units or agencies responding, and take proper personal protection precautions. Ensure that you have a radio, that it works, and that the battery is fully charged. This radio may be your only way to call for help if necessary.

Crime Scenes

EMS practitioners must realize that any type of response could be a potential crime scene. Crime scenes range from motor vehicle crashes (MVCs) to mass murders and may include arson fires, domestic violence, shootings, stabbings, or child abuse. The hazards at a crime scene may be physical, chemical, or biological. All crime scenes have the potential to be dangerous, but active crime scenes have an increased risk, and EMS practitioners, unless members of a Tactical EMS Team, should not be anywhere near an active crime scene. If the call involves a perpetrator who has not yet been apprehended, consider the risk that he or she may return to "finish the job." Whenever possible, move your patient to the ambulance and, if necessary, drive around the corner to a safe location to continue patient care.

IN THE FIELD

Every active crime scene should have boundaries set up to protect EMS practitioners, patients, and bystanders. The boundaries are referred to as zones FIGURE 6-1 . The area where the actual incident is occurring is commonly called the hot zone and should be restricted to allow only essential personnel access because this is the area likely to be the most dangerous. The warm zone may contain a decontamination corridor if any hazardous material exposure due to a weapon is possible. Nonessential personnel, bystanders, EMS, and the media should be located in a perimeter zone, commonly called the cold zone, to ensure that incident actions are not interrupted and safety is maintained. Vehicle, equipment, and personnel staging will also be in the cold zone. The sizes and locations of the zones depend on the incident type.

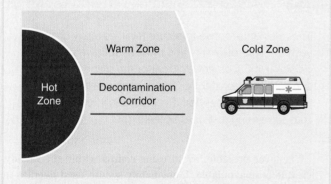

Figure 6-1 The zones of control at a crime scene.
© Jones & Bartlett Learning

The Hazards of Illegal Drugs

While you are driving to an incident, think about the address that dispatch gave. Have any incidents occurred at this address before? If you are responding to a known location where drugs

have been created, sold, or consumed, consider the possibility of booby traps. Booby traps are designed to protect the location and cause serious bodily harm to "intruders." Examples of booby traps include objects falling when doors are opened, holes cut in the center of a hallway floor and covered with a rug, staircase supports removed, and vicious animals that have had their voice box surgically removed.

A person working in a methamphetamine (meth) lab may have been overcome by the highly volatile chemicals used and called EMS for something as routine sounding as difficulty breathing. The chemicals used in the meth lab present many dangers, including inhalation, fire, and explosion hazards.

The Hazards of Alcohol

Dance clubs, bars, and after-hours bars all have the added dangers of alcohol and possibly drugs. The behavior of patients and bystanders under the influence of alcohol or a controlled substance is difficult to anticipate. It is best to have a member of the responding team act as an observer to ensure the safety of those providing direct patient care.

Active Shooter Incidents

As the number of active shooter incidents increases, so does the potential for injury to EMS practitioners. Local policies and procedures will dictate the role of EMS at such incidents. Active shooter incidents are evolving incidents. To save the most lives, triage, hemorrhage control, rapid removal, and rapid transport are needed. To accomplish this, specially trained EMS providers may be working within a casualty collection point close to the hot zone or working with a police escort treating victims as they are found. EMS practitioners who do not have specialized training will be in the cold zone, ready to assess, care for, and transport patients as they are delivered to the cold zone.

IN THE FIELD

Responding to an incident during a civil disturbance may prove dangerous. To many, an EMS practitioner represents authority, and there is a possibility of being attacked by protestors. The mob mentality can cloud even a reasonable person's thought process. A police presence may escalate an incident, so EMS practitioners should load their patient as quickly as possible and leave the immediate area. Working in the back of an ambulance being rocked side to side is not an enjoyable experience.

Secure Facilities

Examples of secure facilities are psychiatric emergency departments, mental health hospitals, jails, and prisons FIGURE 6-2. EMS practitioners frequently transport patients to emergency departments for a psychiatric evaluation and may be called on later to transport a patient to a mental health care facility capable of providing short- and long-term care. Patients with behavioral or mental health concerns are sometimes outwardly violent to EMS practitioners, and practitioners should take appropriate precautions per local policies and procedures to prevent personal injury.

If your agency has a jail, detention center, or correctional facility within its coverage area, it is prudent to know your agency's policies and procedures on how to respond to and operate in these facilities. If no such policy exists, agency heads should meet with site officials to develop policies. A pre-response plan is essential to ensure the safety of EMS practitioners. The level of response, placement of the ambulance on arrival, equipment you are permitted to bring into the facility, and how to safely access the patient are just a few of the procedures that should be agreed on by the EMS agency and facility staff.

EMS practitioners should be prepared for a delay in gaining access to the patient, as well as increased scene time because of security measures. Secure facilities will likely have a specified area for ambulance parking. Make sure you secure the ambulance on arrival.

EMS practitioners risk serious injury if they wear a necktie. The tie can be used to physically manipulate the EMS practitioner and should not be worn. The same goes for a stethoscope around the neck. Common sense would dictate that weapons of any kind not be brought into a secure facility—this includes handguns, knives, and large flashlights. Trauma shears could be a potential weapon, so it is recommended that they be stored in the medical bag and not openly visible.

EMS practitioners will travel through multiple security checkpoints before arriving at the patient. Travel through a secure facility should be only as directed and only with a facility escort. Remain accountable at all times; wandering off could prove dangerous and cause others to have to search for you. In a police station or jail, initial care may be provided in a holding area or cell. Unless there is a mass casualty incident or lockdown, correctional facilities prefer

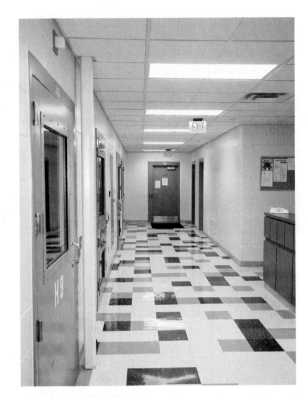

Figure 6-3 Correctional facilities will have transported the patient to the in-house medical center.

Mikael Karlsson/Alamy.

not to have EMS within the prisoner area and will have transported the patient to the in-house medical center FIGURE 6-3.

STAY IN THE FIELD

The rules of response to secure facilities rarely change with the type of facility and must be followed to avoid personal injury or illness. Monitor the scene and your surroundings constantly. Situational awareness is important; pay attention if you suddenly feel uneasy or that something just doesn't feel right.

Whenever possible, avoid using sharps within the facility. When this is unavoidable, immediately secure used needles in the sharps container. Ensure that the sharps container is secured and with you at all times.

Secure facilities may have inmates or residents as "workers" assisting in daily activities. Do not become distracted by this or their offer to assist. Do not allow them to use any of your equipment, including communication devices.

Facility staff is familiar with the rules and regulations that must be followed to ensure safety at all times, and because of this, rarely will EMS be in charge of an incident scene at a secure facility. While within a secure facility, follow the directions of staff, and do not be afraid to ask questions if you are unsure of something.

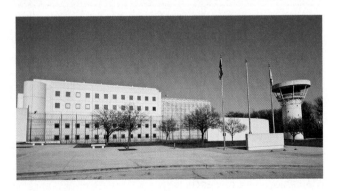

Figure 6-2 A prison is one type of secure facility.

© Benkrut/Dreamstime.com.

Rules of Response to Secure Facilities
- Be aware of your surroundings at all times.
- Lock the ambulance.
- Do not wear anything around your neck.
- Do not bring any weapon into a secure facility.
- Do not carry trauma shears where they are easily visible.
- Do not go anywhere without an escort from the facility.
- Immediately secure all used needles in the sharps container.
- Do not allow any inmate or resident to use your equipment.
- You are in charge of patient care; you are not in charge of the scene.
- Follow directions from staff.
- Notify the hospital before arrival if security is required.

Patients being transported from secure facilities will sometimes require a security presence on arrival at the hospital. Make this notification as early as possible so security is waiting for you when you arrive at the hospital.

Communication Skills during Times of Stress

To understand common signs of escalating anxiety, we must be aware of the powerful emotions present on many EMS scenes. Many of these emotions can be managed with good communication skills. Many of the people we come in contact with during patient care are feeling stress. This stress is caused by anxiety due to the injury or illness and/or fear of the unknown. Usually when there is stress, the body will respond with some form of sympathetic response.

Look and listen for signs of anxiety or agitation. You may hear rapid and/or loud speech. A patient may present with a sarcastic or aggressive tone because he or she is embarrassed. If you notice jaw and/or fist clenching, the tension level the patient is feeling is high. When you add fidgeting, deep and rapid breathing with facial flushing, and a fixed, targeting-type stare, emotions are high, and an attempted assault may take place.

To effectively and safely communicate with patients, family members, and bystanders, EMS practitioners must develop a thorough understanding of verbal and physical or nonverbal communication. How you say something, what you say, and how you look when you say it can affect how the patient responds to you and how much information you are able to elicit. EMS practitioners only get one chance to make a good first impression; solid communication skills will help to ensure a good one.

Imagine for a moment that you are the patient. EMS arrives, and the EMS practitioner begrudgingly enters the scene. He throws his bag on the ground, and, with a heavy sigh while placing his hands in his pockets, he asks why you called for the ambulance. Do you trust this EMS practitioner? Did his attitude make you angry? Do you want to call 9-1-1 back and request another ambulance?

There are already communication barriers that we cannot control, such as differences in age, cultures, and language, and sensory loss in the patient; EMS practitioners do not need to build any additional barriers. Good communication builds trust between the patient and EMS practitioners, and it helps to offset the powerful emotions often present at incident scenes, making assessment and care easier and safer. Poor communication may compromise patient care and put EMS practitioners at risk.

To effectively communicate, EMS practitioners should listen, and not just hear what is being said. One way to show that you are listening is to paraphrase back to the patient what he or she has said.

Nonverbal communication is also a large part of how we communicate with others. The position or stance you take, your body movements, your tone of voice, your facial expressions, and whether you maintain eye contact are all aspects of communication FIGURE 6-4. Words alone do not do the job; your body must say the same thing the words do.

Communication works two ways. EMS practitioners must learn not only to communicate effectively but also to "read" the patient and bystanders around them. Illness and injury can create anxiety and stress, causing a person to act abnormally, responding with a sympathetic "fight-or-flight" response. This can occur at any time during the call. EMS practitioners can prevent possible assaults by being aware of the signs of anxiety or agitation, some of which are increases in the volume of speech, sarcastic or aggressive responses to questions, jaw or fist clenching, fidgeting, fast breathing, and fixed stares. Any action that gives you chills or makes you uneasy should be assessed for possible aggression.

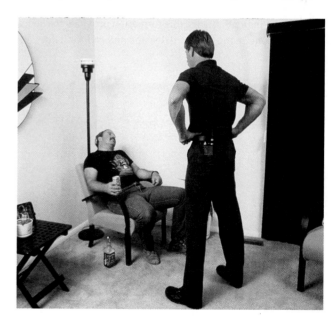

Figure 6-4 Your body language may transmit a completely different message than your words.

© Jones & Bartlett Learning.

Acute stress reactions may manifest in yelling. If patients, family, or bystanders are yelling toward EMS practitioners but not in a threatening manner, allow them to vent; if the EMS practitioners are being threatened, remove yourselves to a safe area. Verbal threats against EMS practitioners are often a precursor to physical violence.

In situations in which the scene is safe and aggression is present or anticipated, EMS practitioners can use verbal deflection, sometimes referred to as verbal judo, to diffuse the situation. Using the correct choice of words, neutralizing insults, responding in kind with compliments, and redirecting the conversation are ways to diffuse a situation. Often verbal aggression can be redirected by explaining everything that you are doing and involving the person in a patient care aspect; making the person a part of the care plan may put him or her at ease.

When practicing verbal deflection and de-escalation, EMS practitioners should adopt the **surveying stance** FIGURE 6-5. The EMS practitioner's body should be slightly at an angle, with the hands above the waist and out of the pockets. The arms should not be crossed or fingers interlaced. The knees should be slightly bent with the weight on the balls of the feet. This is a neutral pose that shows respect to the patient. Maintain eye contact with the patient unless there is a known cultural difference that would require otherwise.

In addition to adopting the surveying stance, EMS practitioners should position themselves in an "L" formation around the patient FIGURE 6-6. This is referred to as the **assessment "L" formation**. This positioning permits one EMS practitioner to address the patient from the front and one EMS practitioner to remain at the patient's side, taking vital signs and performing procedures. The assessment "L" formation gives the patient the illusion of personal space while remaining close enough to maintain a dialogue. The assessment "L" also creates a dilemma in the potentially violent patient: whom and how might the patient attack? If the patient attacks, this formation provides the second EMS practitioner enough time to escape and call for help.

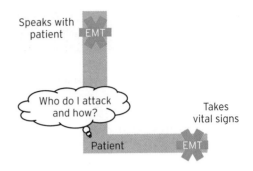

Figure 6-6 The assessment "L" formation.
© Jones & Bartlett Learning.

If a patient attacks, EMS practitioners should yell loud verbal commands like "Stop!" or "Get back!" Yelling will alert bystanders that help is required and will get their attention.

Violence against EMS Practitioners

According to the Experiences with Emergency Medical Services Survey sponsored by the NAEMT, 4 out of 5 EMS practitioners have experienced some form of on-the-job injury. In addition, 52% of EMS practitioners claimed to have sustained injury by assault. Many of the EMS practitioners surveyed expressed that safety is one of their primary concerns.[1]

Unfortunately, assaults against EMS practitioners are far too common. EMS agencies can work to prevent assaults against EMS practitioners by having safety training programs in place, training dispatchers to ask specific questions and give detailed information to EMS practitioners, and having protocols in effect that help EMS practitioners recognize potentially violent situations. In addition, EMS agencies should ensure that their uniforms do not match those of law enforcement; advise members not to enter potentially dangerous situations without law enforcement, and have policies in place that permit and encourage EMS practitioners to leave the scene if violence erupts.

The Six Ds

Likely scenes for violence include those involving the six Ds. Keep in mind that the terms in this mnemonic are only used in this memory tool; these are not diagnostic terms. The six Ds are:

- **Drunk**—It only takes a small amount of alcohol to impair a person's judgment. Larger amounts can lead a patient to become intoxicated and commit uncharacteristic acts of violence. If it is safe to do so, assess the patient to determine if intoxication and not an underlying medical condition, such as hyperglycemia, is the cause of the patient's altered mental status.
- **Drugged**—The patient under the influence of illegal drugs is a serious safety concern for EMS practitioners. Today, EMS practitioners have to deal with patients experiencing unpredictable psychological responses

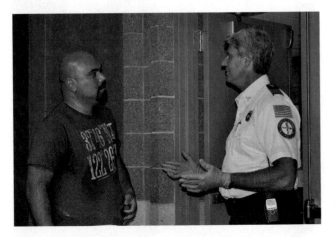

Figure 6-5 When practicing verbal deflection and de-escalation, EMS practitioners should adopt the surveying stance.

Courtesy of Sunstar Paramedics

like extreme anxiety, paranoia, and hallucinations from illegal drugs ranging from meth to bath salts to PCP. Follow local protocols when interacting with patients who may have ingested illegal substances.

■ **Diabetic**—When a patient with diabetes becomes hypoglycemic, very often EMS is called. Without glucose, the brain does not function well, and the patient may even seem to be intoxicated. The patient with hypoglycemia may become violent toward those around him or her, including EMS practitioners. Take appropriate safety precautions and treat the patient as per local protocols.

■ **Deranged**—With a patient experiencing a severe emotional crisis or a psychotic break from reality, safety should be the utmost priority. Carefully observe your surroundings; be especially aware of alternate means of egress, and never put the patient between you and a way out. Keep an observant eye for any weapons or anything that may be used as a weapon. Rule out the possibility of a medical condition as the cause of the patient's behavior. If a behavioral or psychiatric condition is the cause of the patient's extreme responses, your communication skills are critical. Calmly convey the message that you are there to help and not judge or hurt the patient in any way. The louder the patient speaks, the lower your voice should become. Do not tell the patient to calm down; it might only cause him or her to become more agitated. Follow your local protocols and contact law enforcement if you feel that your safety or the safety of others is at risk.

■ **Domestic**—Unfortunately, EMS practitioners encounter domestic violence and the victims involved. You may arrive on a scene while the violence is occurring. As you enter any scene, you should listen for yelling, sounds of a struggle, the breaking of items, and other out-of-the-ordinary noises. If you suspect the possibility of domestic violence during your scene size-up, do not knock on the door or do anything that could alert the perpetrator to your presence. Use the three Rs: retreat to a safe location, radio for assistance from law enforcement, and reassess the situation. If you entered what you consider to be a safe scene, be aware of the bystanders in the room and surrounding rooms because the perpetrator may still be present or might return to the scene while you are still there. Ask all bystanders to vacate the room and ensure that they do not block your egress path. Keep track of where your partner is at all times. Remove the patient to the ambulance as soon as possible.

■ **Desperate**—Desperate patients are not always patients with a long history of behavioral or psychiatric issues; instead, they may be everyday people who are lonely, who feel helpless, and who are unable to endure the pain that they are feeling right now. Desperation may drive some people to perform acts they would not normally do, and this includes violent acts against EMS practitioners. Patients who are experiencing desperation will present with behavioral warning signs such as agitation, yelling, or even making verbal threats. As noted earlier, use your communication skills to de-escalate the tension, follow your local protocols, and contact law enforcement if you feel that your safety or the safety of others is at risk.

IN THE FIELD

Stating or documenting that a patient is "drunk" may be considered slander or libel, and it is not a diagnosis, but more of an assumption. A person who is known to have ingested alcohol may in fact be "drunk," but remember that all medical possibilities of the cause of an intoxicated patient's altered mental status must be ruled out during the patient assessment process.

Patient or Potential Attacker?

The EMS practitioner must be able to distinguish between a patient whose mental status is altered because of a medical emergency and a potential attacker who may be under the influence of drugs or alcohol. When an EMS practitioner is not able to identify a potential attacker, the EMS practitioner may enter a potentially violent scene or remain in a potentially violent scene for too long. A person who verbally threatens or attempts to grab, strike, or spit on the EMS practitioner or who causes the EMS practitioner to feel apprehension or fear is a potential attacker.

Answering a few simple and quick questions will help the EMS practitioner determine if the patient is a potential attacker:

1. *Is this person trying to hurt you?* It seems like a simple question, but all too often EMS practitioners stay too close too long to a potential attacker. Paying attention to "gut feelings" will help an EMS practitioner determine if it is time to leave the scene and call for law enforcement.

2. *Is it this person's intent to do you harm?* Is the patient's behavior intentional because of intoxication or irrational beliefs?

3. *What is your perception?* Are you afraid?

4. *Why is the person threatening you?* Is it confusion due to hypoglycemia or an act of aggression due to intoxication?

5. *Are the words backed up by actions?* If a person is issuing verbal threats while holding a 2×4, the potential for imminent violence is higher than if a prone patient is moaning a verbal threat.

When dealing with a potential attacker, ensure that you have a clear path to exit the scene quickly and use your communication skills to try to de-escalate the situation. Do not argue with the potential attacker, do not order him or her to do anything, and absolutely *do not* attempt to restrain him or her. If you feel this person needs medical attention but is a threat to you, enlist the help of law enforcement to secure the scene. Follow your local protocols on the care and transport in such situations.[2]

IN THE FIELD

The role of EMS practitioners is not to take custody of potential or actual attackers but to provide care to patients. If your safety is in peril, leave the scene immediately and contact law enforcement.[2]

Violent Encounters

Violence against EMS practitioners may or may not involve a weapon. It may come in the form of a verbal attack, physical attack, or a combination of both. Violence against EMS practitioners can be predicted by the actions of the potential attacker. Changes in a person's tone of voice and word choice should be the first clue. This might progress into a verbal assault directed at EMS practitioners and threats of physical harm.

If the situation cannot be defused and a potential attacker begins to make threats of physical violence toward EMS practitioners, then EMS practitioners should be on the lookout for clues that an assault is imminent. The potential attacker might take a fighting stance, clench his or her fists, clench his or her jaw muscles, and have rapid eye movements, flushed skin, and rapid breathing. Any of these physical indicators should prompt EMS practitioners to remove themselves from the immediate scene and take cover or concealment.

Cover and Concealment

Cover or concealment options should become something that all EMS practitioners look for during the scene size-up. **Concealment** hides you from view but does not protect you from projectiles or a potential attacker rushing toward you. A bush would be an example of concealment. **Cover** hides and protects you. A wall, a large tree, and a vehicle are examples of cover.

Reactionary Gap

EMS practitioners should also consider what a minimum safe distance would be, or the proper reactionary gap. The **reactionary gap** is a formula that compares action to reaction, concluding that sudden action is faster than defensive action and that the closer a potential attacker is, the less time an EMS practitioner has to react. If a potential attacker is confirmed to not have a weapon and will not be able to gain access to a weapon, then 6 to 8 feet is a good reactionary gap. Potential attackers with an edged weapon, such as a knife, ice pick, broken bottle, or box cutter, should be given 21 feet as a reactionary gap.

One mile or more should be given as a reactionary gap to potential attackers with a firearm **FIGURE 6-7**. The reactionary gap is like the time, distance, and shielding rule for radiologic emergencies. By increasing the time you have to react, increasing the distance from the potential attacker, and shielding yourself by using cover or concealment, you will layer yourself in protective measures.

Defensive Stance

If an EMS practitioner is met with a violent situation without warning and is unable to rapidly retreat, the EMS practitioner should assume a **defensive stance**. When threatened, the EMS practitioner should do his or her best to create a nonthreatening, nonaggressive appearance. Standing with hands up, with palms forward in an open position, keeping the elbows in, and angling the body 45 degrees to the patient is one option **FIGURE 6-8**.

Weapons

EMS practitioners should have a basic understanding of weapons and how to safeguard them if found during a call or when having to treat a law enforcement officer. EMS agencies should have policies in place regarding the safeguarding of weapons in the field or on the ambulance. As the number of concealed carry permits increases across the country, the likelihood of EMS practitioners finding a weapon while caring for a patient is also increasing. Law enforcement officers and law-abiding citizens who are not affected by an illness or injury causing impairment to their mental state pose little risk. However, those patients who do have an altered mental status and patients with illegal firearms pose a significant safety risk.

EMS practitioners are not in the habit of "frisking" patients for weapons, but they should be looking for them during the physical examination and follow local policies on securing firearms. Patients who are conscious and legally carrying a weapon will most likely tell you that they are armed. Do not permit the patient to hand you a firearm. Even if you are familiar with firearms, do not attempt to unload a gun.

Patients with altered mental status who are armed and patients carrying illegal weapons provide a new and dangerous situation for EMS practitioners. Once a weapon is discovered, the EMS practitioner cannot just ignore it and continue with the assessment and treatment of the patient. If members of law enforcement are on scene, either you or your partner should inform them that a weapon has been found and allow them to secure it safely. If law enforcement is not on scene, follow your local policies, locate a safe means of exit, and contact law enforcement immediately. When treating an injured or ill law enforcement officer, EMS practitioners should allow another law enforcement officer to remove and secure any weapons. As always, follow the training procedures and policies of your agency.

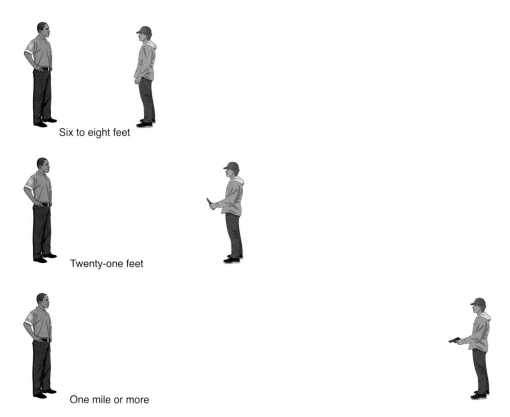

Six to eight feet

Twenty-one feet

One mile or more

Figure 6-7   The reactionary gap for no weapons, an edged weapon, and firearms.
© Jones & Bartlett Learning.

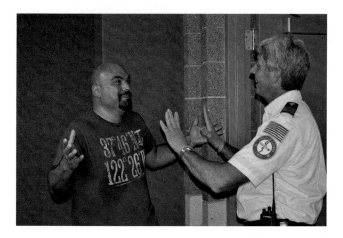

Figure 6-8   To assume the defensive stance, stand with hands up and palms forward in an open position, keep your elbows in, and angle your body 45 degrees to the patient.

Courtesy of Sunstar Paramedics

Excited Delirium Syndrome

Excited delirium (or agitated delirium) is a true medical emergency that can prove to be fatal if not immediately treated. Males are at greater risk for excited delirium. Other risk factors include the use of stimulant drugs, such as bath salts, cocaine, methamphetamine (meth), PCP or LSD, and a preexisting history of schizophrenia or bipolar disorder. Excited delirium onset is acute, and EMS practitioner safety becomes a serious concern. Patients with excited delirium have an increased sympathetic response (fight-or-flight response) and may become agitated, violent, combative, and paranoid. Patients with excited delirium present with psychotic behaviors and may also have hallucinations, have an increase in strength, and become insensitive to pain or self-inflicted injuries.

Suspect excited delirium if the patient is sweating profusely and is hallucinating or presenting with psychotic behavior. Other signs or symptoms EMS practitioners should be observant for are hyperthermia (elevated temperature), tachycardia (rapid heart rate), tachypnea (rapid respiratory rate), hypertension (high blood pressure), and dilated pupils. The patient with excited delirium may be disrobing or have already disrobed prior to your arrival because of his or her extreme body temperature.

IN THE FIELD

Patients with excited delirium do not respond to verbal diffusion tactics. They often have varying mood swings; do not trust the suspected patient with excited delirium who is momentarily calm and cooperative.

The response to a patient with excited delirium should be a tiered, multiagency one. EMS agencies should respond with law enforcement. If EMS practitioners arrive on scene of a suspected patient with excited delirium before the arrival of law enforcement, the EMS practitioners should retreat to a safe area and await their arrival. Policies should be in place regarding the role that each agency will take and what is expected of each agency when dealing with a patient with excited delirium.

Excited delirium may mimic medical conditions that cause altered mental status such as hypoglycemia, psychiatric crisis, and thyroid disorders. Use the AEIOU-TIPS mnemonic to rule out other causes. AEIOU-TIPS stands for:

- Alcohol/acidosis
- Epilepsy
- Insulin
- Overdose
- Uremia
- Trauma
- Infection
- Psychosis
- Stroke

EMS practitioners should follow their local policies regarding the management of patients with excited delirium. If physical restraint is part of local policies, remember that the restraint process is dangerous; the extreme physical exertion may cause cardiac arrest and sudden death in the patient. Never allow your patients to be placed in the prone position, have their extremities tied together, or have excessive pressure put on their backs. These procedures are known to cause *positional asphyxia*, leading to patient death.

Restraining a Patient

EMS practitioners should familiarize themselves with their agency's protocol on the restraint of a patient. EMS agencies should have policies and procedures in effect that have taken into account all local, regional, state, and federal guidelines. The policies and procedures should be reviewed by the agency's legal department. Training of employees should be consistent and ongoing.

Agitated, combative, and violent patients may require some sort of restraint during the prehospital care phase. But remember that we do not attempt to restrain a person who is purposefully violent; that person is not a patient. If needed, police officers would need to take "custody" of that person, and then we could offer care. If restraints are required, every precaution should be taken to ensure the safety of both the emergency responders and the patient. The restraints used should provide some form of dignity to the patient, and you should be able to quickly remove them if patient care dictates it. Patients should never be sandwiched between two devices as a restraint and should never be positioned prone. Both of these methods prevent rapid access to the patient's airway and may cause respiratory compromise

or respiratory arrest. Handcuffs are not medical restraints, and their use is discouraged. Instead, the use of soft restraints is encouraged. If the patient is in custody of police and is handcuffed, a law enforcement officer with a key should ride with the patient.

Patients might continue to struggle even after being restrained. Struggling while restrained may create additional problems for the patient and EMS practitioners. The patient may develop hyperkalemia, rhabdomyolysis, and respiratory or cardiac arrest. Carefully monitor your patient and follow your local policies.

Law enforcement should be requested to the scene, and medical control should be contacted before attempting patient restraint. Ensure that enough trained personnel are available to perform the restraint process safely; usually a minimum of five people is required—one for each limb and one for the head—but six is preferred because someone is needed for the application of the restraint device. If these recommendations cannot be met, it is best to withdraw from the immediate scene and await law enforcement and additional personnel. Be sure to document the incident with as much detail as possible. Begin with your assessment findings, a description of the patient's behavior, any attempts that were made to de-escalate the situation or gain the patient's cooperation, and the restraint method chosen. Be sure to document a continued assessment and monitoring of the patient.

STAY IN THE FIELD

Assisting in restraining a patient can be dangerous for EMS practitioners. It is vital that you maintain your training, follow local policies, and ensure that the proper number of emergency responders is on hand before restraint is attempted.[3]

Restraint Pitfalls

Some of the pitfalls related to application of restraints by EMS practitioners include:

- Lack of individual training
- Lack of cooperative training
- Failure to recognize patients at risk of excited delirium or positional asphyxia
- Failure to report injuries inflicted on EMS practitioners[3]

Errors in Patient Care

Although we would like to think otherwise, medical professionals, including EMS practitioners, are human and do make mistakes. EMS agencies must be cognizant of the fact that errors are inevitable and strive to design and employ systems that minimize the risk to EMS practitioners and their patients. In this section, we discuss several areas that have been identified as being prone to error and discuss ways to minimize the risks.

Medication Errors

According to the Institute of Medicine, each year in the United States, an estimated 7,000 deaths occur because of medication errors.[4] Therefore, it is of utmost importance for EMS agencies and EMS practitioners to use strategies to help reduce and prevent these types of errors. These strategies include the following:

- **Double-check before administration.** Using a system to double-check for accuracy before administration of the medication is known to be a successful method of preventing administration errors. One example is the "5 rights" of medication administration: right patient, right medication, right dose, right route, and right time. Involving a second EMS practitioner in this process increases the chances of success.
- **Ensure competency with dosage calculations.** It is common for EMS practitioners to become complacent with their dosage calculation skills over time. Periodic revalidation of these skills is important for patient safety.
- **Use pediatric resuscitation tapes.** Pediatric dosages for common medications can be difficult to remember because of the lower frequency of exposure to pediatric patients. Use of one of the commercially available resuscitation tapes assists EMS practitioners in determining the patient's weight based on length and provides the correct dosage for the most common medications administered in the field FIGURE 6-9 .
- **Seek uniformity of available supply.** Although this is not always possible, it is beneficial to have uniformity in how medications are supplied. Consistency in concentrations, volumes, and packaging helps to prevent errors in the field.
- **Improve discrimination between "lookalike" medications**. Sometimes a medication has labeling that looks very similar to another medication. One way to

help prevent choosing the wrong medication is to store the "lookalike" medications in different cabinets or drawers within the ambulance or in different sections of the response bag. If these medications absolutely must be stored in close proximity to each other, consider marking one of the boxes or vials with colored tape to distinguish it from the other medication.

Should a medication error occur despite efforts to prevent it, it is important that the environment within the organization encourage reporting. EMS practitioners need to know they can report errors to the hospital and their supervisors without fear of severe discipline. If EMS practitioners feel that their jobs may be in jeopardy, they will be much less likely to report errors, thus placing patients in potential danger. Underreporting of errors also inhibits an EMS agency's ability to discover and address any related problems within their system. EMS agencies that choose to promote a "just culture" within their agency maintain an environment that encourages reporting and supports the parties involved in these situations.

Patient Falls

Depending on the patient care scenario, EMS practitioners may occasionally find themselves in a situation in which it appears that the best decision is to walk the patient to the stretcher. This situation must be approached cautiously because walking a patient to the stretcher poses inherent risks. Assuming that any increased risk to the patient's current health concern has been ruled out, the risk remains that the patient may fall by losing his or her balance, tripping over an object on the floor, or becoming tangled in wires or tubes that he or she may be connected to.

If the patient is to be walked to the stretcher, it is important to ensure that adequate staff are present to assist, the pathway is clear of equipment and other obstacles, and the stretcher is secured in position when the patient attempts to sit down. If the patient uses a cane or walker on a daily basis, this device should be given to the patient to walk to the stretcher. Although the patient is walking under his or her own power, the ambulance crew is responsible for the patient's safety.

Delays in Treatment

EMS practitioners understand very well the importance of performing a thorough patient assessment in an attempt to discover the nature of their patient's illness or injury. If the physical examination of the patient is delayed or is less thorough than necessary, there may be a delay in the formation of a suitable treatment plan.

It is common policy to perform an appropriate patient assessment immediately after making contact with the patient. However, some EMS practitioners may elect not to follow policy on occasion, allowing distractions to interfere with their normal practice and delay the assessment process for certain patients. Some examples include system abusers, sometimes referred to as "frequent flyers," such as intoxicated patients and patients who appear to be

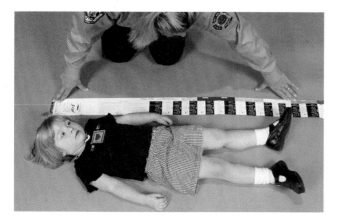

Figure 6-9 Use a pediatric resuscitation tape to avoid errors in patient care.

suffering from mental illness. Often this approach does not lead to a negative outcome for the patient, which serves to reinforce the behavior. Repeatedly delaying the patient assessment or forgoing an appropriately detailed physical examination by taking shortcuts, only to find that it did not make a difference, can cause a shift in what is considered acceptable. This phenomenon is referred to as the "normalization of deviance" and can be very dangerous.[5] As the "deviant behavior" becomes "normalized" and expected within the system, important assessment findings can be missed, potentially leading to negative outcomes for patients.[3]

Equipment Failures

As with many professions, EMS requires its share of specialized equipment. For EMS practitioners to properly care for their patients, they must be able to rely on their equipment. When a critical piece of equipment fails, it can have a devastating impact on the patient's outcome. An EMS practitioner never wants to be treating a patient in cardiac arrest and find that the automated external defibrillator (AED) will not deliver a shock when the button is pushed.

Preventing equipment failures is a function of both the EMS agency and the individual EMS practitioner. Agency responsibilities include:

- Adhering to a preventive maintenance schedule that periodically verifies overall function, calibration, etc.
- Maintaining service records and failure logs.
- Providing adequate backup devices to support the equipment, including batteries and adapters.
- Maintaining an environment that encourages the reporting of equipment problems.

EMS practitioner responsibilities include:

- Checking the equipment at the start of each shift—not simply that it is present, but that it works!
- Following proper procedures such as battery rotation schedules.
- Properly reporting failures or concerns. If possible, details should be provided as to what occurred, when, and under what conditions.
- Maintaining functional knowledge of the equipment. This is especially important if the equipment is not used frequently. By refreshing your knowledge and training, you will prevent "operator error" from being the cause of equipment failure.

Prevention of equipment failure requires a partnership between the agency and EMS practitioners. Working together will reduce the risk of equipment failure and will help protect both the patient and EMS practitioners.

Infections

EMS practitioners often perform their duties in taxing environments, serving diverse patient populations. Illness or injury can affect anyone, and providing care to patients exposes EMS practitioners to many potential infectious diseases.

Preventing infections in the prehospital environment can be challenging. EMS agencies must maintain a comprehensive infection prevention program to ensure a safe work environment for both EMS practitioners and patients.

Personal Responsibility

EMS practitioners should have a heightened awareness for their personal health safety because many illnesses present with the same signs and symptoms. EMS practitioners should continue to follow organizational infectious disease plans even when the underlying disease organism is unknown. Furthermore, consider implementing the following steps on all patient interactions based on the medical direction of Dr. Paul Hinchey of the City of Austin/Travis County EMS System:

- Use the information provided by dispatch to identify patients with symptoms of potentially highly infectious diseases or viruses.
- Maintain a heightened awareness of the potential to interact with patients with new and drug-resistant organisms.
- Limit the number of personnel who have initial contact with the patient by conducting the "view from the door." Such a view can provide the necessary impression that will assist EMS practitioners in determining the need for extensive medical intervention that requires multiple providers. If such an impression is not clearly evident, only one EMS practitioner, in the appropriate PPE, should make patient contact and conduct the patient assessment.
- Obtain a thorough travel history from the patient that covers the past month.
- Wear the appropriate level of PPE based on the mode of transmission of the suspect agent. For example, if you suspect tuberculosis, an airborne disease, don a HEPA respirator **FIGURE 6-10**.

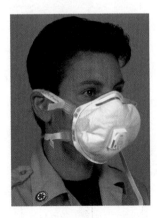

Figure 6-10 Take proper precautions to protect yourself against airborne exposure, including wearing a HEPA respirator.

- For airborne disease, employ PPE to protect against airborne contaminants and droplets.
- Provide surgical masks to all patients with symptoms of a respiratory illness who can tolerate its placement.
- Conduct active surveillance for infected sores, ulcers, lesions, and drainage that may or not be contained by dressings. Specifically examine sites of recent surgical interventions.
- Cover any openings secreting drainage.
- Inquire about the possibility of norovirus when transferring or transporting patients from a facility experiencing cases of acute gastroenteritis.
- Ensure that contact precautions are used during close patient contact. Gowns and masks must be worn along with gloves to prevent contact contamination on your clothing.
- Ensure that the patient is "wrapped" before being moved to minimize environmental contamination.
- Confirm that the hospital or other receiving facilities have been notified of the possibility of an infectious disease.
- Perform thorough cleaning of all equipment that had contact with the patient or the environmental surfaces of the patient's room.
- Ensure safe and prompt usage of an engineered needle system and proper sharps disposal.
- Practice proper hand hygiene diligently.
- If you have a suspicion that a patient may have a new or resistant organism, follow your local organizational procedures for notifying the appropriate public health department so it can undertake the necessary surveillance as soon as possible.

It is vital that any control measures be implemented quickly and sustained to prevent additional transmission. EMS practitioners have been instrumental in assisting in identifying possible infectious outbreaks in the past. For additional guidance on implementing control measures and to report any unusual incidents occurring during any of your agency's responses, contact your local public health department.

WRAP-UP

Summary

- Every emergency scene has the potential to create an unsafe environment for EMS practitioners. Remember that scene size-up is a dynamic, evolving practice, and never take anything for granted.
- Any type of response could be a potential crime scene. All crime scenes have the potential to be dangerous, but active crime scenes have an increased risk. Whenever possible, move your patient to the ambulance and, if necessary, drive around the corner to a safe location to continue patient care.
- While driving to an incident, think about the address that dispatch gave. Have any violent incidents occurred at this address before? Does the address belong to a club or bar where alcohol is served? If the answer is yes, then the risk of violence has just increased, and precautions should be taken.
- Patients from secure facilities with behavioral or mental health concerns are sometimes outwardly violent to EMS practitioners, and practitioners should take appropriate precautions per local policies and procedures to prevent personal injury.
- While within a secure facility, follow the directions of staff, and do not be afraid to ask questions.
- To effectively and safely communicate with patients, family members, and bystanders, EMS practitioners must develop a thorough understanding of verbal and physical or nonverbal communication. How you say something, what you say, and how you look when say it can affect how the patient responds to you and how much information you are able to elicit.
- Poor communication may compromise patient care and put EMS practitioners at risk.

- Communication works two ways. EMS practitioners must learn not only to communicate effectively but also to "read" the patient and bystanders around them.
- Any action that gives you chills or makes you uneasy should be assessed for possible aggression.
- Likely scenes for violence include those involving the six Ds: drunk, drugged, diabetic, deranged, domestic, and desperate.
- EMS practitioners should have a basic understanding of weapons and how to safeguard them if found during a call or when having to treat a law enforcement officer.
- Patients with excited delirium have a fight-or-flight response and may become agitated, violent, combative, and paranoid. They may present with psychotic behaviors and may also have hallucinations, have an increase in strength, and become insensitive to pain or self-inflicted injuries.
- The response to a patient with excited delirium should be a tiered, multiagency one. EMS agencies should respond with law enforcement.
- Agitated, combative, and violent patients may require some sort of restraint during the prehospital care phase. If restraints are required, every precaution should be taken to ensure the safety of both the emergency responders and the patient. Be sure to document a continued assessment and monitoring of the patient.
- EMS practitioners are human and do make mistakes. EMS agencies must be cognizant of the fact that errors are inevitable and strive to design and employ systems that minimize the risk to EMS practitioners and their patients.

WRAP-UP (CONTINUED)

Glossary

assessment "L" formation A formation that permits one EMS practitioner to address the patient from the front and another EMS practitioner to remain at the patient's side, performing patient care. If the patient attacks, this formation provides the second EMS practitioner enough time to escape and call for help.

concealment An object that hides a person from view but does not protect him or her from projectiles or a potential attacker.

cover An object that both hides and protects—for example, a wall, a large tree, or a vehicle.

defensive stance A position that creates a nonthreatening, nonaggressive appearance. The EMS practitioner stands with hands up and palms forward in an open position, keeping the elbows in and angling the body 45 degrees to the patient.

excited delirium A condition in which patients have an increased sympathetic response and may become agitated, violent, combative, and paranoid; they may present with psychotic behaviors and may also have hallucinations, have an increase in strength, and become insensitive to pain or self-inflicted injuries.

reactionary gap A formula that compares action to reaction, concluding that sudden action is faster than defensive action and that the closer a potential attacker is, the less time an EMS practitioner has to react.

surveying stance The body posture to take when defusing a stressful patient encounter. The body is slightly at an angle, with hands above the waist and out of the pockets, arms neutral, and knees slightly bent with the weight on the balls of the feet.

WRAP-UP (CONTINUED)

References

1. National Association of Emergency Medical Technicians. Experiences with Emergency Medical Services Survey; Clinton, MS: National Association of Emergency Medical Technicians; 2005.

2. DT4EMS. How can removing the words "combative patient" reduce workplace violence in medicine? Read this! http://dt4ems.com/?p=643. Accessed September 29, 2015.

3. DT4EMS. Soft restraints = hard times for EMTs, paramedics and nurses. http://dt4ems.com/?p=2403. Accessed September 29, 2015.

4. Institute of Medicine (IOM). *To Err Is Human: Building a Safer Health System*. Washington, DC: National Academy Press; 1999.

5. Banja J. The normalization of deviance in healthcare delivery. *Bus Horiz*. 2010;53(2):139.doi:10.1016/j.bushor.2009.10.006.

Additional Readings

1. DT4EMS, LLC. http://DT4EMS.com.

2. *Guide to Infection Prevention in Emergency Medical Services*. Washington, DC: Association for Professionals in Infection Control and Epidemiology, Inc. (APIC); 2013.

Personal Health

CHAPTER OBJECTIVES

At the completion of this chapter, the participant will be able to:

- Define stress and eustress
- Describe how to recognize stress in yourself, a partner, or a coworker
- Discuss the impact of stress on a person's mental and physical health
- Describe how to improve resiliency skills in order to effectively manage stress

- Describe the importance of rest, relaxation, and sleep
- Discuss the need for physical fitness
- Describe how to plan for appropriate hydration and healthy eating

© Barbol/Shutterstock

SCENARIO

Your kids don't want to go to school today, you can't find your keys, you have no cash, and your significant other took the ATM card. You're now 15 minutes late leaving for work. Your uniform shirt is in the dryer and still damp. If you're late to work one more time, you'll get a written reprimand, which will decrease your merit increase and limit your chances for promotion. But you don't hit any red lights, and you make it to work with minutes to spare.

Your regular partner has called in sick, so you'll be working your 12-hour shift with someone you don't like. The unit is dirty and stocked incompletely. Before you can clean the unit and properly restock it, you get a call on a pediatric trauma code, the result of child abuse. You are unable to successfully intubate the child, and the intraosseous supplies are missing. Upon your arrival at the hospital, the emergency room physician takes you to task for your performance.

1. How many of these events would be stressors for you?
2. How can you keep these events from happening?
3. What strategies do you have in place to help you cope with stressful events?

Introduction

Personal health requires that you be both physically and mentally prepared to deal with the daily issues that life and the job throw at you. This chapter will introduce you to the tools to help you achieve optimal states of physical and mental readiness, as well as information to help you deal with events and conditions that may impair you physically and mentally. Clearly, it is impossible to remove all stressors from your life, but adequate physical and mental preparation can help minimize their impact on you.

Mental Health

Mental health impacts relationships, decision-making abilities, and the capacity to handle stress. Optimal mental health is achieved through a balance of social, physical, spiritual, emotional, and economic states **FIGURE 7-1**. Maintenance of this balance is called homeostasis. When our expectations and experiences do not match, this balance is disrupted, and stress occurs. **Stress** is any event or situation that creates not only an emotional response but also physical and psychological responses. The event is relevant to the person involved and can precipitate an emotional response ranging from anxiety to depression. Physical responses can range from headaches to chronic muscle aches to digestive problems, weight loss, fatigue, and high blood pressure. When stress occurs, the person can perceive the event as harmful, threatening, or challenging.

Not all stress is bad. **Eustress** is positive, beneficial short-term stress. With eustress, psychological balance is restored when a person sees that he or she is capable of tackling life's happy challenges, such as receiving a promotion, getting married, buying a home, having a child, or traveling.

Distress, as in the term "distressing," disrupts a person's psychological balance and can overwhelm him or her physically and mentally. Examples of situations that lead to distress are the

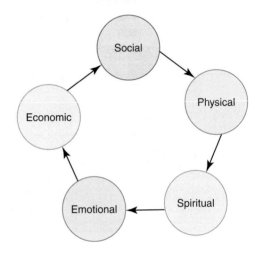

Figure 7-1 Optimal mental health is achieved through a balance of our social, physical, spiritual, emotional, and economic states.
© Jones & Bartlett Learning.

death of a family member, divorce, serious illness or injury of a family member or yourself, financial issues, and challenges with a child's behavior or disability.

Long-term stressors inherent to EMS include a low and/or unpredictable income that makes it difficult or impossible to buy a home, complete a college education, achieve family planning, contribute to children's college funds, or plan for a comfortable retirement. The day-to-day stressors experienced in the EMS workplace include changing schedules, late arrival of next shift coverage personnel, shift start unit checks, and rudeness from coworkers, patients, patients' family members, bystanders, and other healthcare workers **FIGURE 7-2**. On top of this, dispatchers control where we go. We don't control our station and posting locations. All these issues can add up over time and generate levels of discomfort that are stressful.

How often do you experience major and day-to-day stressors on a typical shift? Do you ever feel anxious or depressed?

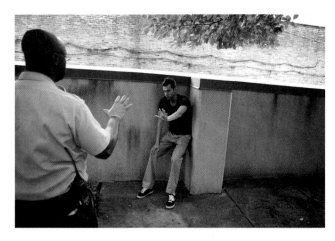

Figure 7-2 EMS is filled with daily stressors, from changing schedules impacted by unexpected or mandated overtime to angry patients.

© Jones & Bartlett Learning. Courtesy of MIEMSS.

Depression and anxiety are comorbid—in other words, they can happen together. We all toss around the words "depression" and "anxiety," but what do they actually mean?

Depression

Depression occurs when a person loses interest or pleasure in living. Common symptoms of persistent sadness and hopelessness may be accompanied by chronic fatigue, tearfulness, and feelings of guilt or worthlessness. A person with depression may lose the ability to concentrate, which makes it more difficult to take an interest in the activities of daily life. There may be changes in body weight from loss of appetite or excessive eating. A person with depression may sleep too much or experience insomnia. Thoughts of death or suicide may intrude into daily activities. Persons with depression may experience deficits in functioning socially.

It is estimated that 20% of the population will experience depression during their lifetime. About three-quarters of people with depression have recurrent episodes.

IN THE FIELD

Depression can place a strain on relationships, and it can increase the likelihood of divorce. It can also impair an EMS practitioner's ability to interact well with partners, patients, and other healthcare providers.

People can become depressed after experiencing events such as a loved one's death or a divorce. Cumulative stress can also trigger depression. When depression persists and causes functional impairment in a person's day-to-day activities, it is called reactive depression.

STAY IN THE FIELD

In 2010, 105 people died from suicide each day in the United States.[1] It has been said that suicide is "a permanent solution to an impermanent condition." If you suspect that your partner or coworker is feeling overwhelmed by life, has confided having such thoughts, or has expressed them on social media, or if you have had such thoughts, bring a supervisor into your circle of trust. There are resources that can help you, a partner, or a coworker regain balance and a sense of purpose. Another option is to contact a resource directly, such as the National Suicide Prevention Lifeline at 1-800-273-8255. Asking for help or obtaining help is not a sign of weakness or betraying a confidence—it is providing life-saving care.

Anxiety

Anxiety is a vague feeling of dread. Physical, emotional, mental, and behavioral reactions can occur simultaneously. Sensations such as queasiness, dizziness, and feeling like your heart is pounding combine with emotions of tenseness, fear, dread, or panic.

Physical signs and symptoms of anxiety include aches, pains, diarrhea, constipation, increased urinary frequency, changes in carbohydrate metabolism, nausea, dizziness, chest pain, tachycardia, loss of sex drive, frequent colds, and irregular menses. Behavioral signs and symptoms may include changes in eating and sleeping habits accompanied by excessive use of alcohol, tobacco, medications, or illegal drugs. Procrastination and social isolation can occur in persons with anxiety. Nervous habits like nail biting or pacing may become evident.

What can we do to deal with these clearly unpleasant feelings? Acknowledging that stressors exist, recognizing the need for help in dealing with the feelings and issues, and asking for help are steps we need to take; how we do that will vary from EMS practitioner to EMS practitioner. Developing resiliency is a good place to start.

Resiliency

Whereas some people seem to be able to quickly accept life's challenges and difficulties, many people need additional training to strengthen their resiliency skills. Resiliency skills enable us to adapt and manage both daily stressors and major life events. The First Response Resiliency course, developed by Michael Marks, Philip Callahan, the Colorado Department of Health Office of Emergency Preparedness and Response, and Centura Health Prehospital Emergency Services, is one such program. It teaches students to develop and improve their resiliency skills to better prepare them to deal with the major stressors that a career in EMS can bring.[2]

In addition to taking the time to recognize stress in ourselves, it is important to communicate well with and be sensitive to the emotional needs of our coworkers. It is part of the culture of safety to be open about sharing difficulties and identifying the times when stress levels are high. Signs and symptoms of stress that are important to note in ourselves and others include anxiousness, difficulty concentrating, being easily irritated, avoiding people and responsibilities, being quick to anger, overreacting, having fatigue, and exhibiting nervous behaviors such as nail biting, pacing, and teeth grinding. Potential physical manifestations of stress include chest palpitations; headaches; digestive problems; muscle tension and pain; disrupted sleep patterns; high blood pressure; weight loss or gain; skin problems such as acne, rashes, and hives; and hair loss.

Other resources to deal with stress include:
- The Code Green Campaign
- American Psychological Association's Road to Resilience
- American Foundation for Suicide Prevention
- American Association of Suicidology
- International Association for Suicide Prevention
- National Suicide Prevention Lifeline at 1-800-273-8255
- 24-Hour Crisis Line at 319-351-3140

Why Is Resiliency Important?

The fatality rate for EMS practitioners is 2.5 times the national average, and EMS practitioners are 3 times more likely to miss work because of injury.[3,4] In addition, because of daily exposure to life-threatening and life-ending events, EMS practitioners are more vulnerable to **posttraumatic stress disorder (PTSD)**, a delayed stress reaction to a traumatic incident. It is estimated that 15 to 20 percent of EMS practitioners experience PTSD.[5] PTSD can increase the risk of alcohol or drug abuse and suicide.

How Do We Address the Problem?

One way to address the problem is to use a program like First Response Resiliency Training, which focuses on promoting

Table 7-1 The 12 Resiliency Skills from First Response Resiliency Training

Physical and behavioral skills	• Goal setting • Proper nutrition • Exercise • Sleep • Relaxation
Cognitive skills	• Perspective • ABCs of our beliefs • Understanding our self-defeating thoughts • Empathy • Dealing with our wins and losses
Social skills	• Reaching out • Social support

12 skills. The 12 resiliency skills are tools that can be pulled from a resiliency toolbox and used as needed. Many of these tools or skills may be familiar, but through First Response Resiliency Training, students learn to apply them systematically to suit their personal needs. Students examine how they have used the 12 resiliency tools in the past and how they might apply them in the future TABLE 7-1.

What's in the Resiliency Toolbox?

The first skills in the resiliency toolbox are the physical and behavioral skills that help provide optimal physical health. To cope well, we need to feel well. The skills are goal setting, healthy eating, exercise, sleep, and relaxation. By integrating these physical and behavioral skills, we are better prepared to deal with stress and utilize the more cognitive and socially oriented resiliency skills.

The cognitive and social skills deal with putting things into perspective, understanding the ABCs of our beliefs, understanding our self-defeating thoughts, practicing empathy, dealing with our wins and losses, reaching out for support, and accessing social support.

Goal Setting

Goal setting is a simple but often overlooked behavioral skill that provides us with a sense of order and control in stressful situations. Knowingly and deliberately setting goals allows us to set a direction. Regular evaluation of our goals and objectives helps us mark progress and make adjustments as necessary. This tool provides us with some degree of control over individual stressors. Setting goals helps us organize our stressors and our responses to them, ideally one stressor at a time.

How do we set a goal? Initially consider the goal to be what you wish to accomplish. The goal needs to be realistically attainable and measurable. The First Responder Resiliency course teaches students to write the goal in a manner that allows them to measure their progress and completion. Students identify the steps necessary to meet the goal so that when all the steps are completed, the goal will be satisfied. Students should develop as many steps as needed to identify key processes in attaining the goal and to mark progress. As each step is completed, it is checked off.

For example, you set for yourself the goal of recognizing the effect of stress on your eating habits. The steps might be to recognize stressors and determine their relationship to what is eaten, when, and how much. This presumes that you have already recognized that you are experiencing stress and that you think it is having an impact on your eating habits because your clothes have become either too tight or too loose.

The next step is to remember a time when students used the goal-setting skill to accomplish a goal. Students write out the past goal statement and the steps used to complete the goal. After examining how the goal-setting tool was used in the past, the First Responder Resiliency course examines how this tool could be applied in the future. Students identify a current issue in their lives and develop a goal and the steps needed to satisfy the completion of the goal. This process of formalizing the skill (writing goals), reflecting on a past experience, and consolidating the skill through practice is the same process used in all the following resiliency skills.

Physical and Behavioral Skills

The balance of resiliency tools under the physical and behavioral skills category includes healthy eating, exercise, sleep, and relaxation. When our bodies are functioning well, we are much more capable of physically and mentally coping with stress.

The physical and behavioral skills build on current baseline measures. Students assess their current physical and behavioral states and identify how a healthier lifestyle could improve these states. Based on the daily requirements of the job, students can determine the steps to take to make positive physical and behavioral changes. For example, changes could include modifying the frequency, intensity, duration, and types of exercise activities to maximize the benefits of routine exercise, reducing health issues related to inactivity as well as the potential for injury.

STAY IN THE FIELD

Overall, positive behavioral and physical adjustments are intended to reduce stress through mindful consideration of eating habits, maintaining a minimal cardiac workout, and obtaining sufficient relaxation and sleep.

Cognitive Skills

The cognitive skills of perspective, understanding our self-defeating thoughts, empathy, and dealing with our wins and losses allow us to mentally cope with stress. In the simplest sense, we might view our interaction with the world as a series of events that lead to consequences or outcomes. Although we cannot control what life throws our way, we can control our reactions to life's events. We can begin by identifying those beliefs that erode our ability to effectively deal with stress and constructing beliefs that better allow us to deal with stress. These more robust and positive beliefs allow us to better put things into perspective and improve our critical thinking skills in difficult situations, and they provide us with better strategies for how we deal with the wins and losses associated with EMS and in life in general.

Social Skills

Because EMS practitioners are those to whom people in great need reach for help, it can be uncomfortable for EMS practitioners to reach out to others for help. There is significant stigma attached to reaching out among EMS practitioners. Among others, the Code Green Campaign is actively working to reduce that stigma. The social skills of reaching out and using our social support networks allow us to establish a safety net for stressful, complex situations in which other individuals can provide insight and support. Research indicates that a strong social safety net is a powerful stress relief mechanism, so it is important for EMS practitioners to improve theirs.

How do we go about developing a social support system? In the First Responder Resiliency course, students start by rating the quality of their current support systems. By identifying their personal needs, students can better select people who can meet their needs.

When applying these concepts in your own life, identify the personal characteristics that you look for in people in your support system. Identify the people you want in your support system and—very important—identify the role each person plays in your support system.

Next, identify the personal characteristics that you provide to your social support system. Identify your strengths and weaknesses. The process of identifying your strengths can help you to become more self-efficacious. **Self-efficacy** is the belief that you are capable of performing in a certain way to achieve a certain goal. For example, if an EMS practitioner was able to remain committed to a diet and exercise program, even during extended weight loss plateaus, he or she could recall that discipline and self-belief and apply it when facing a new life challenge.

Finally, identify the actions that you might use to improve your support system. Always remember that the social support process is very much a two-way street. Consider what *you* can give back to your support system. For example, you can share the resiliency skills you have learned in this chapter, and you can continue to develop your strengths. Also remember that it is far easier to develop a social support system before a crisis occurs.

Resiliency can act as a buffer against developing PTSD, and it can also assist in developing **post-traumatic growth (PTG)**. PTG is an emerging field of study that demonstrates that survivors of trauma can actually grow and become "better people" through their willingness to build greater resiliency skills from the traumas they have confronted. Resiliency skills can empower us to become better caregivers to our patients, families, communities, and, ultimately, ourselves.

Rest, Relaxation, and Sleep

Rest, relaxation, and sleep are important assets in the resiliency toolbox. Exhaustion is a major component of burnout. Sleep does not guarantee that we will be rested or relaxed when we awaken; you cannot rely solely on the quality of sleep to ensure adequate rest. "I had 3 hours of good sleep last night" is an illusion of adequacy. If you don't get 7 to 8 hours of sleep nightly, you are not meeting your physiologic needs. You can't go five or six nights with minimal sleep and make up for it by sleeping 12 hours in one night.

Sleep debt is the difference between the amount of sleep we get and the amount that our bodies need. Physiology doesn't allow us to pay back the sleep debt in a lump sum. Sleep debts impact our behavior and can negatively impact us both physically and mentally by impairing our focus, reflexes, thinking, and social skills.[6]

If the sleep debt is too great, the body will take measures to correct the deficit in the form of microsleeps. During a **microsleep**, the mind ceases to be aware of its surroundings, and the eyes may close for a short period. Microsleeps may last from a few seconds to a few minutes. A microsleep occurring while driving could be fatal **FIGURE 7-3**.

Sleep is also critical for proper brain function. Throughout our waking hours, our brains collect waste products on the

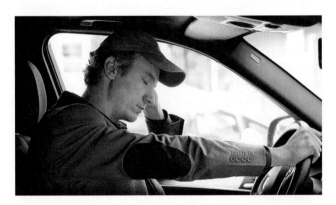

Figure 7-3 Microsleeps are one way the body copes with a sleep debt. Microsleeps can be deadly if they occur while a person is behind the wheel.

© StarsStudio/iStockphoto

cellular level. When we sleep, the brain is able to process these waste products and remove them from the brain.[7,8]

Failure to Sleep

Sleep failure has many causes. Among the causes of sleep restriction or loss are:

- Job-related—24-hour shifts and mandatory overtime
- Personal demands—"My baby has croup."
- Lifestyle choices—"I don't need to be at work until 0800, so I can party until 0200!"
- Sleep fragmentation—Overnight calls
- Disruptions to the body's clock—Jet lag, night shifts, or alternating day/night shifts
- Use of sedating medication—Antihistamines or cough suppressants
- Untreated sleep disorders—Sleep apnea

How to Get a Better Night's Sleep

First, try to obtain a regular sleep schedule. Avoid caffeine and alcohol before bedtime. Don't eat an hour to an hour and a half before bedtime. Keep your bedroom comfortable by maintaining a suitable temperature, masking outside noises, and keeping the room as dark as possible. Daytime sleepers should silence telephones and related devices. Heavy curtains or room-darkening shades may be needed to block out daylight **FIGURE 7-4**.

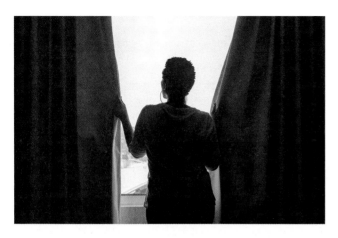

Figure 7-4   If you must sleep during the day because of shift work, light-blocking curtains can help create more ideal sleeping conditions.

© davidf/iStockphoto

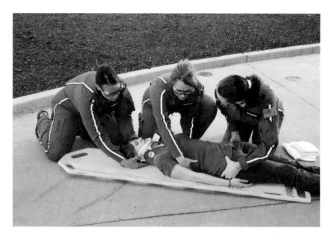

Figure 7-5   An EMS practitioner will bend, twist, reach, and pull repetitively throughout the shift.

© National Association of Emergency Medical Technicians.

Fitness and Health

Physical fitness is a requirement of being an EMS practitioner. Overall fitness is not determined solely by the amount of weight that a person can lift. An EMS practitioner must be able to bend, twist, reach, and pull repetitively in a manner that hurts neither the EMS practitioner nor the patient FIGURE 7-5. As an EMS practitioner, you need to have the functional strength, stability, and mobility to tolerate the stresses imposed on your body on a daily basis.

Fitness is a critical component of overall physical and mental wellness, in addition to being able to meet the physical requirements of the job. Regular physical activity, healthy eating, and stress reduction all improve overall wellness. An essential step in achieving fitness is addressing any body weight issues.

Society's current obesity crisis is reflected within the EMS community. According to a study published in the journal *Obesity* in 2009, over 75% of recruits for the fire and EMS services were either overweight or obese.[9]

Currently the body mass index (BMI) classifies the ranges for normal, overweight, and obese weights. The BMI itself is a formula of weight divided by height. See FIGURE 7-6 for a current BMI chart that lists the weight ranges for each category.

Another metric to use is waist circumference. Carrying excess weight in the abdomen increases the risk of contracting several life-threatening diseases. To reduce the risk of heart disease, some types of cancer, and diabetes, a woman's waist should be less than 35 inches and a man's less than 40 inches.

The two most powerful tools in the weight control toolbox are diet and exercise. Let's explore how to use these tools in our daily lives.

Exercise Guidelines

When designing or refining a personal exercise program, it is a good idea to consult with local trainers to assist you. You can also consult the publication "Task Performance and Health Improvement Recommendations for Emergency Medical Services Practitioners" produced by the American Council on Exercise (ACE) for the National Association of Emergency Medical Technicians. This publication is designed to provide general exercise guidelines for EMS practitioners. The ACE program focuses on improving the EMS practitioner's mobility, in addition to strength and cardiovascular training, to prevent injuries that can occur while performing daily activities.

According to Gray Cook, MSPT, OCS, CSCS, the movements performed during daily activities can be broken down into five patterns: bending/raising and lifting/lowering movements (e.g., standing up from a chair); single leg movements (e.g., running); upper body pushing movements (e.g., pushing a stretcher); upper body pulling movements (e.g., pulling a stretcher closer); and rotational movements (e.g., twisting at the waist) FIGURE 7-7A-E.[10] To avoid injury, ACE recommends that EMS practitioners:

- Perform exercises that train the five basic movement patterns at least two days per week
- Perform moderate-intensity cardiorespiratory physical activity such walking 150 minutes a week, or
- Perform 75 minutes of intense cardiorespiratory physical activity (such as running) a week[11]

Remember that you can be creative and fit exercise into your daily routine. Each time you complete a transport, perform one stretch on the back of the ambulance FIGURE 7-8. This will keep your body loose and primed for the next call. Simple activities, such as doing step-ups and push-ups on the back of the ambulance between calls, burn calories. Every little bit of exercise adds up!

BMI Height	19	20	21	22	23	24	25	26	27	28	29	30	31	32	33	34	35
												Weight in Pounds					
4'10"	91	96	100	105	110	115	119	124	129	134	138	143	148	153	158	162	167
4'11"	94	99	104	109	114	119	124	128	133	138	143	148	153	158	163	168	173
5'	97	102	107	112	118	123	128	133	138	143	148	153	158	163	158	174	179
5'1"	100	106	111	116	122	127	132	137	143	148	153	158	164	169	174	180	185
5'2"	104	109	115	120	126	131	136	142	147	153	158	164	169	175	180	186	191
5'3"	107	113	118	124	130	135	141	146	152	158	163	169	175	180	186	191	197
5'4"	110	116	122	128	134	140	145	151	157	163	169	174	180	186	192	197	204
5'5"	114	120	126	132	138	144	150	156	162	168	174	180	186	192	198	204	210
5'6"	118	124	130	136	142	148	155	161	167	173	179	186	192	198	204	210	216
5'7"	121	127	134	140	146	153	159	166	172	178	185	191	198	204	211	217	223
5'8"	125	131	138	144	151	158	164	171	177	184	190	197	203	210	216	223	230
5'9"	128	135	142	149	155	162	169	176	182	189	196	203	209	216	223	230	236
5'10"	132	139	146	153	160	167	174	181	188	195	202	209	216	222	229	236	243
5'11"	136	143	150	157	165	172	179	186	193	200	208	215	222	229	236	243	250
6'	140	147	154	162	169	177	184	191	199	206	213	221	228	235	242	250	258
6'1"	144	151	159	166	174	182	189	197	204	212	219	227	235	242	250	257	265
6'2"	148	155	163	171	179	186	194	202	210	218	225	233	241	249	256	264	272
6'3"	152	160	168	176	184	192	200	208	216	224	232	240	248	256	264	272	279

Locate the height of interest in the leftmost column, and read across the row for that height to the weight of interest. Follow the column of the weight up to the top row that lists the BMI. A BMI of 19 to 24 is in the healthy range, a BMI of 25 to 29 is in the overweight range, and a BMI of 30 and above is in the obese range. Due to rounding, these ranges vary slightly from the NHLBI values. A calculator for adult BMI is available at http://www.nhlbisupport.com/bmi. A child and adolescent BMI calculator is available at http://apps.nccd.cdc.gov/dnpabmi.
Source: Reproduced from US Departments of Agriculture and Health and Human Services. *Dietary Guidelines for Americans*. 6th ed. Washington, DC: US Government Printing Office; 2005.

Figure 7-6 BMI chart.

Reproduced from U.S. Departments of Agriculture and Health and Human Services. *Dietary Guidelines for Americans*. 6th ed. Washington, DC: US Government Printing Office; 2005.

STAY IN THE FIELD

To stick to your exercise plan, you should first plan and then record your daily workouts.

STAY IN THE FIELD

The so-called diet beverages have been related to increased cardiovascular morbidity and mortality. Some found that surprising. An exact mechanism has not been described. One postulate suggests that artificial sweeteners change the gut bacteria, which has metabolic consequences. Another speculates that the tongue is an "energy sensor," and the sweet taste fools the brain into anticipating an energy source. The taste without the fuel is thought to disrupt normal cerebral mechanisms of appetite control.[12]

A Healthy Diet

Water is the best choice for hydration in a healthy diet. We assess the hydration status of our patients as a matter of routine. Do we ever think about our own personal hydration? If we wait until we are thirsty, we are already short of water. The need to urinate about every 90 minutes is an indicator of adequate hydration.

If we attempt to rehydrate with caffeinated and sugary beverages, we can become dehydrated because of the diuretic effect. If we stay dehydrated long enough, we can experience electrolyte imbalances that can make us prone to muscle spasms and infections.

Plan to meet your hydration needs on the job by bringing water in a container that can be easily stored and secured in the ambulance. Remember to practice healthy hydration habits off-duty as well. If you do not develop and practice healthy hydration habits at home, you will be unlikely to follow them at work. The same consideration applies to your food intake.

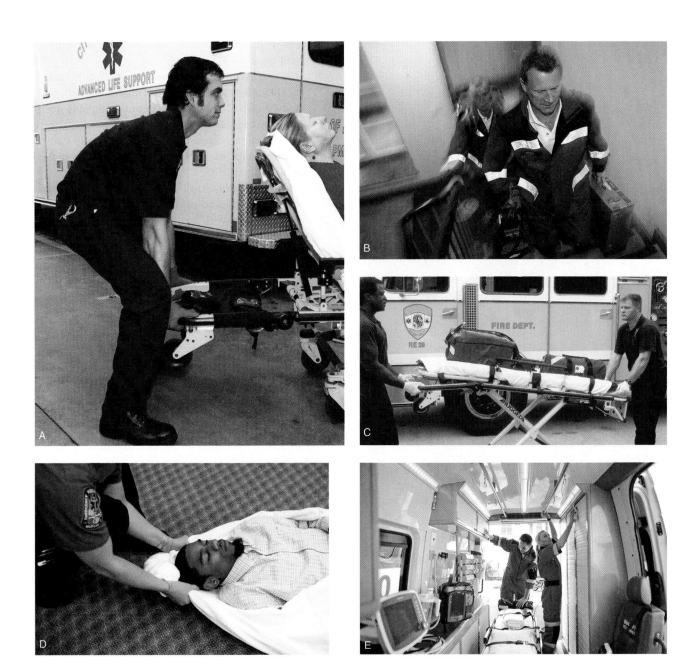

Figure 7-7 There are five movements performed during daily activities. A. Bending/raising and lifting/lowering movements. B. Single leg movements. C. Upper body pushing movements. D. Upper body pulling movements. E. Rotational movements.

A. © Jones and Bartlett Learning. Courtesy of MIEMSS; B. © Jochen Tack/imageBROKER/age fotostock; C. © Jones & Bartlett Learning. Courtesy of MIEMSS; D. © Jones & Bartlett Learning. Courtesy of MIEMSS; E. © Zero Creatives/Corbis

Meal Planning

Making healthy food choices is challenging enough when you are at home with a refrigerator full of fresh fruits and vegetables. Obtaining healthy food choices while you are on duty is an even greater challenge. Set yourself up for success by preplanning and bringing healthy meals with you.

Today's education on nutrition suggests eating foods from the six main food groups in the right amounts based on your age, gender, and activity level. For example, a moderately active woman between the ages of 19 and 30 requires around 2,000

calories per day, whereas a moderately active man requires about 200 calories more.

Of the six food groups, the current advice is:

■ *Fruits.* Eat a variety of fruits; choose fresh, frozen, canned, or dried fruit. Go easy on fruit juices. Read labels; corn syrup should be avoided altogether. Look for products that have no sugar added.
■ *Vegetables.* Vary the vegetables you eat; eat more dark green vegetables and orange vegetables, as well as

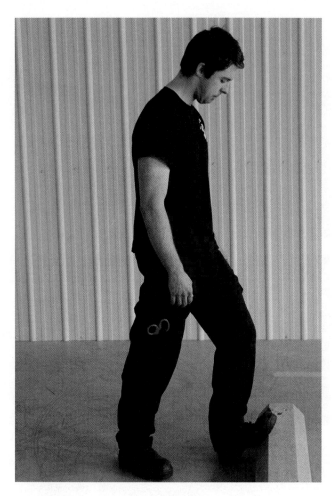

Figure 7-8 Stretching between calls will keep you limber and ready.
© Bryan Fass. Used with permission.

dried beans and peas. Half of your plate should be fruits and vegetables.

- *Grains.* Make half your grains whole. Whole grains are healthier because they contain important nutrients that reduce the risk of disease. They also contain more protein and more fiber. Consume 3 ounces of whole-grain bread, cereal, crackers, rice, or pasta every day. Look for the word "whole" before the grain name on the list of ingredients.
- *Meat and beans.* Go lean on protein; choose low-fat or lean meats and poultry. Bake, broil, or grill. Vary your choices with more fish, beans, peas, nuts, and seeds.
- *Dairy.* Eat calcium-rich foods, choosing low-fat or fat-free items.
- *Fats.* Know your fats; make most fat sources from fish, nuts, and vegetable oils. Limit solid fats like butter, stick margarine, shortening, and lard.

Finally, it is a good idea to check the amount of sodium in canned and prepared foods; choose those with lower amounts.

WRAP-UP

Summary

- Mental health impacts relationships, decision-making abilities, and the ability to handle stress. Optimal mental health is achieved through a balance of social, physical, spiritual, emotional, and economic components.
- Stress is any event or situation that creates not only an emotional response but also physical and psychological responses. When stress occurs, the person can perceive the event as harmful, threatening, or challenging.
- Eustress is positive, beneficial short-term stress. With eustress, psychological balance is restored when a person sees that he or she is capable of tackling life's happier challenges, such as getting married or buying a home.
- Distress disrupts a person's psychological balance and can overwhelm him or her physically and mentally. Distress includes losing a family member or experiencing a serious illness or injury.
- Long-term stressors inherent in EMS include a low and/ or unpredictable income.
- The day-to-day stressors experienced in the EMS workplace include handling changing work schedules and enduring rudeness from others.
- Depression occurs when a person loses interest or pleasure in living. A person with depression may lose the ability to concentrate, which makes it more difficult to take an interest in the activities of daily life.
- Anxiety is a vague feeling of dread. Physical, emotional, mental, and behavioral reactions can occur simultaneously. Procrastination and social isolation can occur in people with anxiety.
- Resiliency skills enable people to adapt and manage both daily stressors and major life events. Courses such as the First Response Resiliency course teach students to develop and improve their resiliency skills.
- The first skills in the resiliency toolbox are the physical and behavioral skills that help provide optimal physical health. The skills are goal setting, healthy eating, exercise, sleep, and relaxation.
- Sleep and relaxation are important assets in the resiliency toolbox because exhaustion is a major component of burnout.
- Sleep debt is the difference between the amount of sleep we get and the amount that our bodies need. Unfortunately, we cannot pay back the sleep debt in a lump sum. Sleep debts impact our behavior and can negatively impact us both physically and mentally.
- Physical fitness is a requirement of being an EMS practitioner. An EMS practitioner must be able to bend, twist, reach, and pull repetitively in a manner that hurts neither the EMS practitioner nor the patient. As an EMS practitioner, you need to have functional strength, stability, and mobility to tolerate the stresses imposed on your body on a daily basis.
- Fitness is a critical component of overall physical and mental wellness, in addition to being able to meet the physical requirements of the job. Regular physical activity, healthy eating, and stress reduction all improve overall wellness.

WRAP-UP (CONTINUED)

Glossary

anxiety A vague feeling of dread accompanied by activation of the autonomic nervous system to produce both physical and mental sensations ranging from dizziness to panic.

depression The loss of interest or pleasure in living.

distress A disruption of a person's psychological balance that can overwhelm him or her physically and mentally.

eustress Short-term stress that is positive and beneficial; psychological balance is restored when a person sees that he or she is capable of tackling life's happy challenges.

microsleep When the mind ceases to be aware of its surroundings and the eyes may close for a short period; it may last from a few seconds to a few minutes.

post-traumatic growth (PTG) An emerging field of study that demonstrates that survivors of trauma can actually grow and become "better people" through their willingness to build from traumas they have confronted.

self-efficacy The belief that you are capable of performing in a certain way to achieve a certain goal.

sleep debt The difference between the amount of sleep you get and the amount that your body needs.

stress Any event or situation that creates an emotional response.

References

1. Centers for Disease Control and Prevention, National Center for Injury Prevention and Control. Web-based Injury Statistics Query and Reporting System (WISQARS) [online]. (2010). [cited October 19, 2012]. Available from http://www.cdc.gov/injury/wisqars/index.html.
2. Gunderson J, Grill M, Callahan P, Marks M. Responder resilience. *JEMS*. 2014;39(3): 57–61.
3. Maguire BJ, Hunting KL, Smith GS, Levick, NR. Occupational fatalities in emergency medical services: a hidden crisis. *Ann Emer Med*. 2002;40:625–632.
4. Maguire BJ, Smith S. Injuries and fatalities among emergency medical technicians in the United States. *Prehosp Disaster Med*. 2013;28(4):376–382.
5. Beaton R. Extreme stress: promoting resilience among EMS workers. *Northwest Public Health*. 2006;23(2).
6. Butkowski TJ. Sleepy and unfit. *Safety + Health*. 2014;189(6): 66–67.
7. Benedict C, Cedernaes J, Giedraitis V, et al. Acute sleep deprivation and neurodegeneration. *Sleep*. 2014;37(1):195–198.
8. Nedergaard M. Garbage truck of the brain. *Science*. 2013;340(28): 1529–1530.
9. Tsismenakis AJ, Christophi CA, Burress JW, Kinney AM, Kim M, Kales SN. The obesity epidemic and future emergency responders. *Obesity*. 2009;17(8):1648–1650.
10. Cook G. *Athletic Body in Balance*. Champagne, IL: Human Kinetics; 2003.
11. American Council on Exercise. *Task Performance and Health Improvement Recommendations for Emergency Medical Service Practitioners*. San Diego, CA: ACE; 2012.
12. Kirkwood C. Tricking taste buds but not the brain: artificial sweeteners change brain. September 5, 2013. http://blogs.scientificamerican.com/mind-guest-blog/tricking-taste-buds-but-not-the-brain-artificial-sweeteners-change-braine28099s-pleasure-response-to-sweet/. Accessed May 20, 2015.

Suggested Reading

1. American Council on Exercise. *Task Performance and Health Improvement Recommendations for Emergency Medical Service Practitioners*. San Diego, CA: ACE; 2012.
2. Leiter MP, Maslach C. Conquering burnout. *Scientific American Mind*. 2015;26(1):30–35.
3. Murray CJL, Lopez AD, eds. *The Global Burden of Disease: A Comprehensive Assessment of Mortality and Morbidity from Diseases, Injuries and Risk Factors in 1990 and Projected to 2020*. Cambridge, MA: Harvard University Press; 1996.
4. Wehrenberg M, Prinz S. *The Anxious Brain*. New York, NY: W.W. Norton and Company; 2007.
5. Rothbaum B. *Pathological Anxiety: Emotional Processing in Etiology and Treatment*. New York, NY: Guilford Press; 2006.
6. Gotlib I, Hammen C. *Handbook of Depression*. New York, NY: Guilford Press; 2002.
7. Beaton R. Extreme stress: promoting resilience among EMS workers. *Northwest Public Health*. 2006;23(2):8–9.
8. Gist R, Taylor VH, Raak S. White paper: suicide surveillance, prevention, and intervention measures for the US Fire Services. Presented at: The Suicide and Depression Summit hosted by the National Fallen Firefighters Foundation. July 11 to 12; 2011; Baltimore, Maryland.
9. Callahan P, Marks MW, Grill M, Wiemokly G. *First Response Resiliency*. OneTreePsych; 2013.

CHAPTER 8

Conclusion

CHAPTER OBJECTIVES

After reading this chapter, the participant will be able to:

- Identify the organizations that are working to help improve and promote a culture of safety within EMS

- Describe how each EMS practitioner can take personal responsibility for making the work environment safer

© Barbol/Shutterstock

SCENARIO

You and your partner have had a busy shift and are returning to quarters. You're driving in moderate traffic and discussing after-work plans when your cell phone rings. Glancing down at the phone, you see that it's your spouse calling. As you reach down to pick up the phone, you hear your partner exclaim, "Red light, red light, RED LIGHT!" Halfway through the intersection, you hear metal on metal when a vehicle hits your ambulance on the passenger side, is driven across the intersection, and suddenly lurches to a stop. When the airbags deflate, you look over to see your partner unconscious, bleeding from the head, while you are dangling upside down, held in place by your seatbelt.

1. What is your first responsibility when driving an ambulance?
2. How should this type of distraction be handled?
3. What is your next action?

Introduction

How we behave on every call impacts our safety, our patients' safety, and the safety of the community at large FIGURE 8-1. If we drive too fast for the current road conditions, we put all the ambulance occupants and the general public at risk of injury. If we don't buckle our seatbelt before the ambulance starts moving, our patients will notice. Such behaviors are observed and assessed by the public. When members of the public see EMS practitioners engaging in unsafe behaviors, they may deem it appropriate to engage in the same unsafe behaviors. The status of the overtly unsafe EMS practitioner may diminish the profession in the eyes of the public, who may be less likely to follow instructions from caregivers they do not respect.

In addition to modeling safe behaviors, we must create an environment in which respect among our colleagues is a given. Good communication will not occur without respect. Lapses in communication may prevent vital information from being

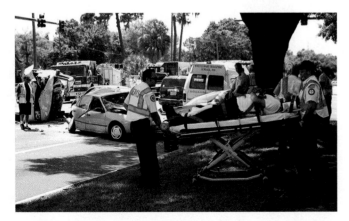

Figure 8-1 How you behave on every call impacts your safety, your patients' safety, and the safety of the community at large.

© ZUMA Press, Inc./Alamy

IN THE FIELD

Good management practices must be embraced by those who develop them and by those who perform them on a daily basis. In addition, adequate resources must be supplied for the workforce to function safely. Finally, the workforce must adhere to safety policies and use the resources supplied by management.

shared. As Chapter 2: *Crew Resource Management* discusses in detail, the chain of survival applies to each of us. If one of us is unsafe, all of us are unsafe.

As EMS practitioners, we must be active regarding, educated on, and well practiced in all facets of safety. When it comes to safety, there is no room for "that's not my job." In addition to having the skills obtained from mandatory safety training, we must be perceptive, recognize new hazards, and actively engage in mitigating those hazards. For example, the Centers for Disease Control and Prevention (CDC), in concert with the Assistant Secretary for Preparedness and Response (ASPR), issued a "Detailed Emergency Medical Services (EMS) Checklist for Ebola Preparedness." During our initial training, how many of us were trained on hemorrhagic viruses that originate in Africa? What a perfect example to illustrate that we must be continually vigilant and communicative!

As EMS practitioners, we must be open to change and constructive criticism. Shared ignorance benefits nobody. Join professional organizations and participate in their activities. Subscribe to professional journals to enhance your awareness of what other EMS professionals experience.

Engage in dialogue with other professionals, not just those in EMS. Do you think that public health officials, infectious disease specialists, design engineers, or risk managers/engineers may have information from which you could benefit? We cannot limit the scope of our perspective to EMS. Other medical professionals have access to information that is not EMS specific but is vital for us to know. The risks from new infectious diseases or the enhanced risks from old ones are first recognized in the public health and infectious disease arenas, often well in advance of their emergence as EMS issues. Engineers have knowledge that can affirm or refute the practicality of ideas that EMS practitioners have regarding ambulance design.

Significant Steps in Creating an EMS Culture of Safety

Ambulance

The ambulance is your place of business FIGURE 8-2 . As such, it must be designed in such a fashion that it can be used safely. This is such a critical issue that organizations such as the Commission for the Accreditation of Ambulance Services (CAAS), the National Fire Protection Association (NFPA), and the U.S. General Services Administration (GSA) have developed design standards for ground ambulances, which include the Ground Vehicle Standard for Ambulances (GVS-2015), NFPA 1917, Standard for Automotive Ambulances, and KKK-A-1822F. It is wise to familiarize yourself with these standards because different agencies will follow a specific standard based on their affiliation.

The intended performance of the ambulance is the basis for the design standards. The design standards factor in the environmental conditions in which the vehicle will be used, such as weather and terrain. The external structure is designed to protect occupants from the impact of external forces. The roads and traffic flow are considered in determining the best mechanical design.

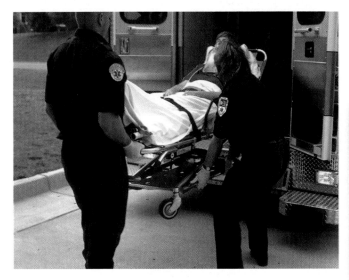

Figure 8-2 The ambulance is your mobile office.
© Jones & Bartlett Learning. Courtesy of MIEMSS.

The internal structure of the ambulance should be free from sharp edges, protrusions, and any other hazards. The design of the patient care compartment should be based on the movements required for EMS practitioners to provide patient care. EMS practitioners should be able to reach both the equipment and the patient while wearing proper restraints. This promotes operational efficiency as well as safety.

The driver and all ambulance occupants must have restraint systems proved to safely secure them and a solid structure in the ambulance to absorb potential traumatic forces. Design engineers consider the worst case scenarios, such as rollovers and high-speed crashes, when creating the structural and restraint system designs.

IN THE FIELD

The concept that the ambulance is your office mirrors the idea that EMS is a business. In some cases, it is a business in which profit is not a goal. However, the cost of operations is a critical component that must be evaluated for the survivability of any EMS system. How much does it cost to run and maintain an ambulance for an average transport? What is the ambulance replacement cost? The agency's managers must apply the same level of intensity to fiscal efficiency as EMS practitioners do to clinical efficiency in the field.

An interdisciplinary approach to ambulance design brings engineers, manufacturers, salespeople, purchasers, and EMS practitioners together. Technological advances in multiple arenas occur concurrently, so keeping information in professional silos is unproductive. For example, unless a design engineer receives input from an EMS practitioner, how will the design engineer know how large to make a space for the securement of a defibrillator?

STAY IN THE FIELD

Just as emerging technologies partially shape the standards of care, nonclinical technologies partially shape the standards of safety. Computer-aided dispatch, global positioning systems (GPS), and onboard monitoring systems continue to advance in complexity and effectiveness. However, we must understand that no technology is a panacea. It must be used in a thoughtful and systematic manner.

NAEMT

The National Association of Emergency Medical Technicians (NAEMT) EMS Workforce Committee influences the operational standards of EMS systems through the development of professional standards for EMS in position papers. NAEMT position papers demonstrate the unity of the goals within the EMS community as a whole and the needs of EMS practitioners. The acquisition of resources by EMS systems for the protection and safety of EMS practitioners is more likely to occur when the importance of safety is called out as a common goal for the EMS profession to achieve.

NAEMT also expresses the importance of safety through the development of continuing education courses, such as EMS Safety, which was developed to address the unacceptable levels of injury and illness seen among EMS practitioners.

EMS Safety Foundation

Safety issues for ambulance personnel are not confined to the United States. The EMS Safety Foundation uses a professional staff to collect, evaluate, and distribute the results of ambulance safety research efforts from all over the world. For example, safer ambulance designs used in Europe became widely available in America because of the EMS Safety Foundation's efforts.

Federal Regulations

The awareness of the dangers to which EMS practitioners and all first responders are exposed when responding to emergencies on highways led to federal legislation requiring emergency responders to wear high-visibility safety vests. Although the legislation on the wearing of these vests focused on federal highways, the federal government's emphasis on the importance of safety vests as a key tool in preventing injury and deaths in first responders resulted in their use becoming commonplace on all roadways. Remember, "When your feet are on the street, the vest is on your chest."

STAY IN THE FIELD

Safe EMS practitioners have longer and more comfortable careers. It is easier to function and stick around if you are healthy and uninjured!

International Association of Fire Chiefs

The impact of sleep deprivation on safety is so critical that the International Association of Fire Chiefs (IAFC) issued a report entitled "The Effects of Sleep Deprivation on Fire Fighters and EMS Responders" and developed an educational program to address this issue.[1] The results of the IAFC's efforts could alter the EMS system's approaches to current scheduling structures and the number of hours that EMS practitioners are allowed to work.

EMS Culture of Safety
Safety Begins with You

You will not be safe unless you come to work mentally and physically prepared every day. This takes planning, preparation, and discipline. Without a "sound mind in a healthy body," you will not be able to effectively process the information in your work environment. You will not recognize the potential dangers. What you do not recognize, you cannot share. This places you and your coworkers in harm's way.

IN THE FIELD

Share what you've learned in this book. You do not have to give a formal lecture; you can instruct your coworkers through your safety-conscious behaviors.

Do not engage in unsafe behaviors, and do not tolerate them in others. When you see hazards, act FIGURE 8-3. Immediately communicate the presence of the potential hazards to anyone in the area who may be harmed. Take immediate action to minimize the impact of the unsafe conditions and inform your management team as necessary.

Do not get lulled into a false sense of security. Analyze your behaviors and those of your coworkers, not just individually but collectively. Talk with your peers and think out loud with each

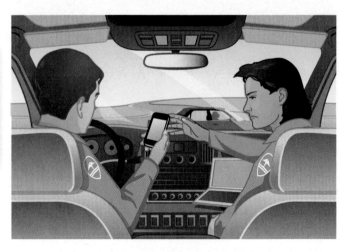

Figure 8-3 If you see a potential hazard, speak up! Warn others and take action to eliminate the hazard.

other. It can be as simple as, "We should have moved the table before we moved the patient." Or it could be, "We need new wiper blades right now. Call dispatch."

Promote formal reporting processes. Incident reports can be used to identify hazards, quantify them, and monitor trends. Near-miss reporting, or the recognition of hazardous events that almost happened but did not, helps to identify results based on simple luck as compared with those based on good preventive practices. Near-miss reports can provide crucial insights that can be used to develop safety practice standards. If your EMS system has a safety committee, be an active member on it, or at least provide input to the committee.

Continuous learning will keep your mind open to new ideas. Open-mindedness will allow you to evaluate new ideas objectively. Use critical reasoning when presented with proposed design changes in vehicles and equipment. Do not reject or accept anything solely on the basis that it is new.

Constantly think about ways to make your workplace safer, share them with your coworkers, and submit them to management. When it comes to safety, do not forget that little things matter too. Do you need more lighting in the garage? Are the steps slick? Does the station keep running out of hand sanitizer in the bathroom?

STAY IN THE FIELD

Emergency vehicle operators should always drive the ambulance safely, without distraction, and ambulance crew members should require anyone who drives them to behave in the same manner.

IN THE FIELD

What are some things we can do today, tomorrow, next week, and next month to keep building the EMS culture of safety?

- Talk the talk: talk to others in your EMS system about what you have learned and how it can apply to them and the EMS system.
- Walk the talk (or drive the ambulance):
  - Use what you have learned to lead by example. Be a safe EMS practitioner.
  - Get some sleep!
  - Put your phone away.
- Lead the charge:
  - Talk with your superiors and let them know the benefits of creating a safer work environment and the dangers of *not* doing so.
  - Participate in "near-miss" (close calls) and crash reviews.
  - Join your EMS system's safety committee.
- Keep up to date:
  - Use the *EMS Safety* text as a reference for the future.
  - Read the increasing number of articles on EMS safety topics in the major EMS and fire service magazines.
  - Join an online EMS Safety discussion group.
  - Sign up for alerts from EMS World, JEMS, and EMS1.
  - Continue your NAEMT membership (when you take the EMS Safety course, you will receive a free one-year online membership).
- Be open to new ideas:
  - Major design changes may be proposed in our vehicles and equipment. Evaluate the changes objectively, and be an advocate for those changes that will benefit you and your EMS system.
  - Think of ways to make your workplace safer, and submit ideas to your supervisors; do not just talk about them.
- Become an instructor for EMS Safety and share the information you have learned with your EMS system and other EMS agencies in your region.

WRAP-UP

Summary

- How we behave on every call impacts our safety, our patients' safety, and the safety of the community at large.
- When members of the public see EMS practitioners engaging in unsafe behaviors, they may deem it appropriate to engage in the same unsafe behaviors.
- Safety depends on good communication. Good communication occurs in an environment where everyone is respected.
- As EMS practitioners, we must be active, educated, and well practiced in all facets of safety. In addition to the skills obtained from mandatory safety training, we must recognize new hazards and actively engage in mitigating them.
- As EMS practitioners, we must be open to change and constructive criticism. We can enhance our awareness of what other EMS professionals experience by joining professional organizations, subscribing to professional journals, and speaking with a diverse range of professionals, from public health workers to ambulance engineers.

- NAEMT influences safety in EMS through the development of professional standards for EMS in position papers and through the development of continuing education courses, such as EMS Safety.
- Do not engage in unsafe behaviors, and do not tolerate them in others. When you see hazards, act.
- Do not get lulled into a false sense of security. Analyze your behaviors and those of your coworkers, not just individually but collectively.
- Incident reports can be used to identify hazards, quantify them, and monitor trends. Near-miss reports can provide crucial insights that can be used to develop safety practice standards.
- Continuous learning keeps our minds open to new ideas. Open-mindedness allows us to evaluate new ideas objectively.
- All EMS practitioners should constantly think about ways to make our workplaces safer. Ideas should be shared with coworkers and submitted to management. Safety is both an individual and group effort.

Reference

1. International Association of Fire Chiefs. Sleep deprivation. http://www.iafc.org/sleep. Accessed May 28, 2015.

Scene Safety for Infectious Diseases

Understanding the Risks of Communicable Disease

To maintain personal safety, understand what diseases a patient can transmit to EMS practitioners. Assisted living and long-term care facilities can expose practitioners to gastrointestinal outbreaks such as noroviruses and *Clostridium difficile*, as well as interaction with multi-drug-resistant organisms like methicillin-resistant *Staphylococcus aureus* (MRSA) and carbapenem-resistant *Enterobacteriaceae* (CRE). Safety concerns regarding communicable diseases also extend back to the patient who may be predisposed to infections because of immune compromise, comorbid illnesses, and trauma.

EMS practitioners should understand the risks of communicable disease that the community presents. The demographics and activities of the community can be used to identify the means by which certain diseases may become present in the community. EMS practitioners should be aware of the activities that the business, education, and entertainment communities provide for individuals who travel from locations where endemic or new emerging diseases have been identified. Such activities include educational seminars, conventions, sporting events, and music festivals that bring participants from multiple countries. The increasing practice of medical tourism, in which individuals travel to locations specifically for invasive surgical procedures, presents the opportunity for the introduction of and exposure to newly identified resistant organisms.

Personal Responsibility

Safety begins even before responding on incidents. Ensuring proper protection against the most common infectious diseases through up-to-date immunizations is the first step. Maintaining a healthy body through good nutrition, adequate sleep, and mechanisms for stress relief will make the EMS practitioner a less susceptible host for many infections.

Before each duty shift, EMS practitioners should undertake a self-assessment of their health, including whether they have a fever; exhibit signs of respiratory illness such as nasal congestion, runny nose, sore throat, or cough; or exhibit signs of gastrointestinal illness, such as nausea, vomiting, diarrhea, and extreme discomfort from excessive gas. They should also conduct a body examination for any nonintact skin or open wounds.

STAY IN THE FIELD

Carefully consider when to shave to ensure adequate time for the development of scabs and healing in the case of an accidental "nick"; this will prevent an inadvertent portal of entry for a patient's body fluids.

Any open nonscabbed wounds should be covered with a dressing and bandage to prevent contamination. Should the self-assessment reveal a gastrointestinal problem, the ill EMS practitioner should remain at home until he or she has been without symptoms for 48 hours. If a respiratory infection is suspected, such as influenza, EMS practitioners should remain at home until at least 5 days have passed since the start of symptoms and the fever has not been present for at least 24 hours.

The Five Bs

Given the multitude of communicable diseases, it is difficult for an EMS practitioner to remember them all. To assist in determining the disease risks a patient can present, EMS practitioners should focus on the mechanisms for exposure and the infectious fluids associated with each. One method that EMS practitioners can use to assess each patient for the risk of infectious diseases is the five Bs concept: blood, breath, bowels, bodies, and bugs TABLE A-1 . Grouping diseases by body systems, functionality, and interactions should assist in identifying the disease risk to EMS practitioners. If EMS practitioners know what they are potentially facing, they can take appropriate precautions.

Table A-1 **The Five Bs**				
Blood	**Breath**	**Bowels**	**Bodies**	**Bugs**
HIV	Tuberculosis	Norovirus	MRSA	Scabies
Hepatitis B	Pertussis	Salmonella	Lesions	Bed bugs
Hepatitis C	Influenza	*E. coli*	Rashes	West Nile virus
Anthrax	Meningitis			Chikungunya
	Measles			Dengue
Viral hemorrhagic fevers	SARS	*Clostridium difficile*		
	MERS			

Blood

The risk to EMS practitioners from bloodborne pathogens became most apparent with the identification of the human immunodeficiency virus (HIV) in the early 1980s. While other bloodborne pathogens were recognized before HIV, the significance of such exposures was not as obvious. EMS practitioners now are aware of the risks from hepatitis B and C as well.

STAY IN THE FIELD

The term *bloodborne pathogen* does not pertain just to contact with blood and all its components but also to semen, vaginal secretions, cerebrospinal, synovial (a viscous fluid that lubricates the joints of the fingers, shoulder, elbow, and hip), and amniotic fluids, as well as breast milk. Urine, sweat, and feces are not considered infectious unless visibly contaminated with blood.

Although there still should remain high awareness for HIV, with the availability of drug therapy and ongoing disease monitoring, the risk of infection from patients with HIV has decreased significantly. Rather than interacting with patients with HIV for their underlying immunological condition, now EMS practitioners are more apt to interact with patients with HIV during more routine medical emergencies such as cardiac and trauma events. The number of occupational sero-conversions related to patients with HIV or AIDS has remained very stable, with no new reports since 1999. Of the approximately 200 confirmed and possible sero-conversions, only 13 have involved EMS personnel.[1]

The greatest risk of exposure to bloodborne pathogens is through a needle stick with a contaminated device. The highest risk for infection from hepatitis B in the unvaccinated EMS practitioner is between 6% and 30%; the risk for hepatitis C is 1.8%; and the risk for HIV is 0.3%.[2]

Breath

The risks associated with breathing present in one of two ways: through large droplets that allow organisms, such as meningitis, pertussis (whooping cough), and seasonal influenza, to adhere to the watery surface when expelled during coughing and sneezing, and through the mucous membranes of the eyes, nose, or mouth. The risk for exposure to such diseases is greatest when the EMS practitioner is within 6 feet of the patient.

The second way is through contact with smaller particles, usually 5 micron in size or smaller, that may stay airborne within the environment for an extended period and can be inhaled by the EMS practitioner during patient interaction, as in the case of tuberculosis and measles. Such diseases can also be found on droplets and may infect the EMS practitioner through the droplet route.

EMS practitioners should maintain heightened awareness when confronted with any patient presenting with an acute febrile respiratory illness, which may include fever plus one or more of the following: nasal congestion, runny nose, sore throat, or cough. Many illnesses present with the same signs and symptoms, so it is important to continue to follow respiratory infectious disease precautions even when the underlying disease organism is unknown.

Special attention should be given when responding to group living settings such as halfway houses and jails. EMS practitioners should be alert when confronted with patients who have fevers of unknown origin, individuals who have a serious illness with a decreased level of consciousness, foreign-born persons, and homeless individuals. EMS practitioners should also consider the time of year and its associated disease presentations.

Such awareness should be more acute during the initiation of aerosol-generating and resuscitation procedures such as nebulized respiratory treatments, endotracheal intubation, open suctioning of airways, and cardiopulmonary resuscitation, which can frequently result in the presence of a large amount of body fluids, such as saliva and vomit.

Bowels

The risks to EMS practitioners associated with the gastrointestinal system involve contact with organisms that will create gastroenteritis. The typical presentation is nausea, vomiting, diarrhea, and extreme discomfort in the form of gas and cramping. A number of organisms cause these symptoms. Among the most notable are norovirus, *Clostridium difficile*, commonly referred to as C. diff, *E. coli*, and Salmonella. Deaths from such infections continue to increase, with the vast majority of deaths caused by *Clostridium difficile*. The second leading cause is the norovirus.[3]

Given the underlying medical conditions for many patients, the majority of such gastrointestinal illnesses are contracted in hospitals and long-term care facilities. EMS practitioners should be more attentive to patients who present with gastroenteritis symptoms while in such facilities and take appropriate precautions even if the initial response was for something other than gastroenteritis. Additionally, EMS practitioners should be alert when there are increased responses to the same facility for patients with the same signs and symptoms.

Bodies

It is important for EMS practitioners to be attentive to lesions and rashes on the body surface of patients. These lesions can exude fluids that can provide for the transmission of organisms such as MRSA. Such attention should be through active surveillance during the patient assessment process. Identifying sores and lesions can assist in determining if there is a potential communicable disease present. Initiating barrier protection in the form of contact precautions will prevent inadvertent contamination to EMS practitioners.

Bugs

The risks of disease from contact with insects are very low for EMS practitioners. The usual concerns involve more of the unsightliness of some of the infestations encountered in the prehospital setting. Among the most common are scabies and bed bugs. The nature of prehospital work activities can result in EMS practitioners participating in active emergency responses as well as physical and continuing education training during the hours that mosquitoes and other disease-carrying insects are most active. Such activities can increase the potential exposure to mosquito- and tick-borne diseases such as West Nile virus, encephalitis, eastern equine encephalitis, St. Louis encephalitis, California encephalitis, and Powassan encephalitis. EMS practitioners should be attentive during physical training and emergency activities and wear long pants and long-sleeved shirts when outdoors, particularly at dawn and dusk. Use an approved insect repellent every time you go outside, and follow the instructions on the label.

Scabies are mites: small, brownish, flattened insects that feed solely on the blood of the host on which they reside. Scabies are found in folds of skin, particularly on the fingers, elbows, and genitalia. Such infestations continue to appear with increasing frequency. Scabies do not transmit disease from the host to the EMS practitioner. Contracting scabies requires intimate, close contact that most commonly occurs during the movement of the patient from his or her bed to the associated ambulance stretcher. If an EMS practitioner becomes infested, treatment is available for such significant exposures.

Bed bug infestations do not indicate a lack of general hygiene or cleanliness of the patient. Bed bugs are mostly active at night because they remain close to where they feed and take on the sleeping schedule of the host. Just as with scabies, transmission of other diseases is highly unlikely. The most important consideration when confronted with a possible bed bug infestation is the placement of equipment. Maintaining a distance from the primary source of the infestation and keeping equipment bags closed and sealed will diminish the potential for the inadvertent contamination of the equipment bag with bed bugs.

EMS practitioners should also be attentive to patients who have returned from areas where there are increased mosquito-borne disease transmissions, such as dengue, chikungunya, and other hemorrhagic fever viruses. With evidence of a dengue outbreak occurring in Puerto Rico and its continued transmission in Key West, Florida, travel to certain domestic locations may also have posed a risk for the patient.[4] EMS practitioners should consider such potential diseases when evaluating patients returning from dengue-affected areas—both domestic and abroad—who present with an acute febrile illness within 2 weeks of their return. Such information can be obtained by inquiring about any travel within the past month of symptom onset.

Personal Protective Equipment

An essential component of utilizing personal protective equipment (PPE) is the consistent use of proper hand hygiene. Ensuring proper hand hygiene before and after the application of all PPE will diminish the opportunity for the inadvertent exposure via the mucous membranes, such as rubbing tired eyes with your hands. Remember, the use of equipment does not replace basic hygiene measures such as handwashing.

PPE is used to protect EMS practitioners and patients by preventing potentially infectious microorganisms from contaminating your hands, eyes, and clothing and being transmitted to others. PPE reduces, but does not completely eliminate, the possibility of acquiring an infection. PPE is only effective if used correctly. The purpose of PPE is to create a barrier between the patient and the EMS practitioner.

For EMS practitioners, PPE includes any combination of nonsterile examination gloves, eyewear such as goggles, face shields, or safety glasses, impervious gowns, surgical/procedure masks, and fit-tested N95 masks. EMS practitioners should consider the application of PPE according to the needs of the situation and specifically when there is significant contact with patient or environmental surfaces, a demonstrated need for eye and respiratory protection (especially during any airway management procedures), or equipment cleaning.

EMS practitioners should not don PPE until they initiate patient care. Premature application of PPE can result in damage to the structural integrity of the PPE as well as environmental contamination transferred to the patient.

This damage can create a false sense of protection when in fact there has been a compromise of the PPE to the point of leading to inadvertent inoculation.[5]

Once EMS practitioners have completed patient care, they should properly remove their PPE, with attention to preventing inadvertent cross-contamination. The PPE should be placed in the appropriate container for disposal. After the removal of all the PPE, appropriate hand hygiene should be initiated using soap and water or hand rubbing with an alcohol-containing hand cleaner.

Precautions

Once the risk for exposure is identified, EMS practitioners should don the approprirate PPE. EMS practitioners should consider the need for a combination of precautions that may be used on patients who are infected with diseases that have multiple routes of transmission. There are four types of precautions: standard precautions, droplet precautions, airborne precautions, and contact precautions.

Standard precautions, previously known as universal precautions or body substance isolation (BSI), are intended to be applied to the care of all patients in all healthcare settings regardless of the suspected or confirmed presence of an infectious agent. According to the Healthcare Infection Control Practices Advisory Committee (HICPAC) of the Centers for Disease Control and Prevention:

> Standard precautions are based on the principle that all blood, body fluids, secretions, excretions except sweat, non-intact skin, and mucous membranes may contain transmissible infectious agents.[6]

By utilizing the term *standard precautions*, all medical practitioners have the same understanding of the level of precaution that has been initiated. Implementation of standard precautions constitutes the primary strategy for the prevention of healthcare-associated transmission of infectious agents among patients and healthcare personnel.

According to HICPAC:

> The application of Standard Precautions during patient care is determined by the nature of the provider-patient interaction and the extent of anticipated blood, body fluid, or pathogen exposure. For some interactions (e.g., performing venipuncture), only gloves may be needed; during other interactions (e.g., intubation), use of gloves, gown, and face shield or mask and goggles is necessary.[6]

Often in emergency medicine, the causes or infections are not readily apparent. This increases the need to be attentive when interacting with patients who exhibit respiratory symptoms.

Droplet precautions are to be used in addition to standard precautions for all individuals presenting with an acute febrile respiratory illness, which may include fever plus one or more of the following: nasal congestion or runny nose, sore throat, or cough and/or individuals known to have a respiratory-droplet-spread disease, such as *N. meningitides*, pneumonic plague, and pertussis. In addition to following standard precautions, EMS practitioners should wear a surgical/procedure mask when within at least 3 feet of the infected individual, and the patient should wear a surgical/procedure mask if tolerated.

Airborne precautions should be employed if the infectious agent is spread via an airborne vector, which forms small particles that may remain airborne for an extended period. Examples include tuberculosis, measles, chickenpox, smallpox, and pandemic illness.

According to HICPAC:

> Additionally, certain procedures can also impact transmission of infectious agents by producing aerosols. These are deemed "high risk respiratory procedures" and include intubation, extubation, deep tracheal suctioning, and nebulized respiratory treatments. A fitted N95 mask is recommended for any "high risk respiratory procedure" in the setting of suspected acute febrile respiratory illness.[6]

Contact precautions should be used when the organism is transmitted by direct contact with the patient or contaminated environmental surfaces. Such precautions should be initiated with patients with large infected ulcers and drainage that is not contained by dressings. Examples of such organisms inlcude any drug-resistant organism, *Clostridium difficile*, scabies, *E.coli* O157:H7, and noro-type viruses.

Exposure Management

It is hoped that most EMS practitioners will go their entire career without experiencing an occupational exposure to an infectious disease. However, even a solid awareness of the five Bs of infection may not be enough to prevent an EMS practitioner from experiencing such an occupational exposure.

STAY IN THE FIELD

Such exposures can be very stressful and create some apprehension as the EMS practitioner navigates through the follow-up process, which can be as long as 6 months. It is important for all EMS practitioners to know the appropriate process for the evaluation, follow-up, and treatment related to any suspected occupational exposures for their agency.

Contact with an infectious agent in and of itself does not result in the development of an infection. To become infected requires an appropriate portal of entry, an adequate amount of the infectious agent, and a susceptible host. For bloodborne pathogen exposures, the transmission risk increases if the injury is deep, if there is evidence of visible blood on the device, if the device was placed in a vein or artery, and if the source patient has indication of a high viral load of the infectious organism.

Regardless of the degree or significance of the exposure, the importance of rapid action in the event of potential exposure cannot be overemphasized. Should the evaluation of the exposure indicate that postexposure prophylaxis (PEP) is warranted, such PEP needs to be initiated within hours.

For HIV, the sooner the better, but the PEP becomes less effective 24–36 hours after the exposure. Should the source patient be later found to be negative, PEP can be discontinued.

For those unvaccinated or nonresponders to the hepatitis B vaccine, hepatitis B immunoglobulin (HBIG) must be administered within less than 7 days of the exposure, preferably within 24 hours. If the source patient is hepatitis C positive, there is currently no PEP treatment, but ongoing monitoring and follow-up are essential.

It can be more difficult to determine if an EMS practitioner has been exposed to a repiratory disease such as meningitis, tuberculosis, or pertussis. Even with a suspicion at the time of patient contact, testing and follow-up will take time. Many times, exposure is not known until later because materials from the source patient must be cultured to see if an organism can be grown.

Additionally, special situations may prolong the investigation and final disease determination of the source patient. Examples of such situations include patients who are unconscious, unwilling to consent to testing, or pronounced dead on-scene or shortly after arrival at a medical facility; exposures to an unknown source due to improperly discarded contaminated medical sharps; and events that occur off-duty.

Insect infestations usually do not require postexposure treatment. If exposure to scabies is significant, treatment with a miticidal medication that kills the scabies mite can be considered.

Safety Needle Systems

Because the greatest risk for acquiring an occupational exposure is through a contaminated needle or other medical sharps, EMS practitioners should have available injury protection devices, such as self-sheathing catheters and syringes, as an intregal part of all such medical sharps. EMS practitioners should ensure proper knowledge on the use and activation of such devices, and the devices should not adversely impact the delivery of patient care or result in EMS practitioners delaying treatment; in addition, no one should attempt to circumvent the intended safety functions of the device. EMS practitioners should ensure that all contaminated medical sharps are properly disposed into a puncture-resistant container.

Cleaning and Disinfection

Equipment and evironmental surfaces can provide a mechanism for the spread of infectious diseases from one patient to another and to other EMS practitioners. To prevent such mechanisms, it is important to ensure that all contaminated equipment is properly cleaned and disinfected for the next emergency response. Once all the associated patient care needs have been addressed, the EMS practitioners should return to the ambulance for cleaning and disinfection.

It is vital that EMS practitioners use a disinfectant rated to kill the targeted bacteria, viruses, and other microorganisms on nonliving surfaces. EMS practitioners should refrain from using antiseptic soaps, which only inhibit the growth and development of microorganisms and are typically used on the skin and mucous membranes. Although such antiseptics may be derived from disinfectants, the concentrations are not strong enough to adequately eradicate the organism. Currently, approved disinfectants are adequate in the cleaning and disinfection of the usually encountered organisms. Special cleaning and disinfection is not warranted unless specific recommendations are issued for newly emerging or resistant strains of organisms.

Before commencing with cleaning and disinfection, EMS practitioners should don the appropriate PPE such as gloves, mask, and eyewear to minimize contact with dispersed contaminated materials and potential inadvertent exposure. EMS practitioners should consider cleaning with disposable towels to minimize cross-contamination and laundering issues.

Using approved cleaning and disinfection agent(s), EMS practitioners should wipe down the stretcher frame, mattress, hand rails, and any other potentially contaminated stretcher mechanisms. EMS practitioners should make sure they remove all organic material such as blood, other bodily fluids, and dirt from the equipment. All patient care equipment used on the patient should be thoroughly cleaned before being placed back into the ambulance. Once the equipment has been adequately and totally cleaned, a disinfectant in the appropriate concentration and for the specified contact time should be applied and allowed to air dry.

After cleaning the equipment and removing all PPE, the EMS practitioner should initiate appropriate hand hygiene once again with an alcohol-containing hand cleaner. EMS practitioners are once again ready for additional ambulance responses.

Summary

EMS practitioners should have a heightened awareness of personal health safety because many illnesses present with the same signs and symptoms. EMS practitioners should continue to follow organizational infectious disease plans even when the underlying disease organism is unknown. Furthermore, consider the following steps on all patient interactions:

- Use the incident information provided by dispatch that alerts EMS practitioners to a possibly symptomatic patient.
- Maintain a heightened awareness of the potential for interface with patients with new and resistant organisms.
- EMS practitioners should limit the number of personnel who have initial contact with the patient by conducting the "view from the door." Such a view can provide the necessary impression that will assist in determining the need for extensive medical intervention requiring multiple EMS practitioners. Should such an impression not be clearly evident, only one responder, in the appropriate PPE, should make patient contact and conduct the initial patient assessment.
- Obtain a thorough travel history that covers the past month.
- Wear the appropriate level of PPE based on the mode of transmission of the suspect agent.
- Where respiratory vectors are considered, employ PPE in accordance with airborne and droplet precautions.
- Provide surgical masks to all patients with symptoms of a respiratory illness who can tolerate their placement.
- Conduct active surveillance for infected sores, ulcers, lesions, and drainage that may or may not be contained by dressings. Specifically examine sites of recent surgical or other invasive interventions.
- Cover any openings exuding or secreting drainage.
- Inquire about the possibility of norovirus when transferring/transporting patients from a facility experiencing cases of acute gastroenteritis.

- Ensure that contact precautions are used during close patient contact. Gowns and masks must be worn along with gloves to prevent contact contamination on clothing.
- Ensure that the patient is "wrapped" before being moved to minimize environmental contamination. Such wrapping should have the patient covered with a clean sheet with the sides and ends tucked under him or her. Additional coverings should be applied to ensure that all areas that may be touched during transport are covered adequately.
- Confirm that the hospital or other receiving facilities have been notified of the possibility of an infectious disease.
- Perform thorough cleaning of all equipment that had contact with the patient or the environmental surfaces of the patient's room.
- Ensure safe and prompt usage of an engineered needle system and proper sharps disposal.
- Understand the need for diligence in hand hygiene.
- If you have a suspicion that a patient may have a new or resistant organism, follow organizational procedures for notifying the appropriate public health department so officials can undertake the necessary surveillance as soon as possible.

References

1. Joyce MP, Kuhar D, Brooks JT. Occupational acquired HIV infection among health care workers–United States, 1985–2013. *MMWR*. 2014;63:1245–1246.
2. Centers for Disease Control and Prevention. Updated U.S. Public Health Service guidelines for the management of occupational exposures to HBV, HCV, and HIV and recommendations for postexposure prophylaxis. *MMWR*. 2001;50(RR11);1–42.
3. Lessa FC, Mu Y, Bamberg WM, et al. Burden of *Clostridium difficile* infection in the United States. *N Engl J Med*. 2015; 372:825–834.
4. Centers for Disease Control and Prevention. The Dengue Update. http://www.cdc.gov/dengue/dengue_upd/resources/Dengue UpdateVo3No1.pdf. Accessed June 22, 2015.
5. Centers for Disease Control and Prevention. Infection Control. http://www.cdc.gov/oralhealth/infectioncontrol/faq/protective_ equipment.htm. Accessed June 22, 2015.
6. Siegel JD, Rhinehart E, Jackson M, Chiarello L, Healthcare Infection Control Practices Advisory Committee. *2007 Guideline for Isolation Precautions: Preventing Transmission of Infectious Agents in Healthcare Settings*. Atlanta, GA: Centers for Disease Control and Prevention; 2007.

Additional Readings

1. Garner JS, Hospital Infection Prevention Practices Advisory Committee. Guideline for isolation precautions in hospitals. Centers for Disease Control and Prevention. *Infect Control Hosp Epidemiol*. 1996;17:53–80.

2. Occupational Safety and Health Administration. OSHA Fact Sheet: OSHA's bloodborne pathogens standard. https://www.osha.gov/SLTC/bloodbornepathogens/index.html. Accessed June 22, 2015.

3. Centers for Disease Control and Prevention. Recommendations for preventing transmission of human immunodeficiency virus and hepatitis B virus to patients during exposure-prone invasive procedures. *MMWR*. 1991;40(RR08):1–9.

4. The Association for Professionals in Infection Control and Epidemiology. *Guide to Infection Prevention in Emergency Medical Services*. Washington, DC: APIC; 2013.

5. Centers for Disease Control and Prevention. Immunization of health-care personnel: recommendations of the Advisory Committee on Immunization Practices (ACIP). *MMWR*. 2011; 60(RR07):1–45.

GLOSSARY

aggressive driving Operating a vehicle with aggressive actions, without concern for other drivers.

anxiety A vague feeling of dread accompanied by activation of the autonomic nervous system to produce both physical and mental sensations ranging from dizziness to panic.

assessment "L" formation A formation that permits one EMS practitioner to address the patient from the front and another EMS practitioner to remain at the patient's side, performing patient care. If the patient attacks, this formation provides the second EMS practitioner enough time to escape and call for help.

cachectic Possessing an appearance of wasting away; usually associated with poor nutrition or disease.

challenge More direct than an alert; when a team member physically moves into the action circle, prepared to take the next step of emergency intervention.

cognitive distractions Distractions that take the emergency vehicle operator's mind off the road and operation of the vehicle.

coherence When truth aligns with some specified set of sentences, propositions, or beliefs.

complacency What occurs when you believe you are so good at your job that you stop thinking about how to do it properly.

concealment An object that hides a person from view but does not protect him or her from projectiles or a potential attacker.

conflict resolution A range of processes aimed at alleviating or eliminating sources of conflict; generally includes negotiation, mediation, and diplomacy.

conspicuity The ability of a vehicle to draw the attention of other drivers.

cover An object that both hides and protects—for example, a wall, a large tree, or a vehicle.

crew resource management (CRM) A tool originally instituted by the airline industry in 1980 to optimize performance and outcomes by reducing the effect of human error through the use of all available resources.

defensive stance A position that creates a nonthreatening, non-aggressive appearance. The EMS practitioner stands with hands up and palms forward in an open position, keeping the elbows in and angling the body 45 degrees to the patient.

depression The loss of interest or pleasure in living.

direct costs Payments made to physicians, rehabilitation professionals, insurance carriers, and attorneys; compensatory salaries for lost work; and employee replacement costs.

distress A disruption of a person's psychological balance that can overwhelm him or her physically and mentally.

due regard When driving in emergency mode, the emergency vehicle operator should give regard and attention to everyone else sharing the road.

engineering controls Changes made to the work environment through the use of equipment to avoid work-related injury.

eustress Short-term stress that is positive and beneficial; psychological balance is restored when a person sees that he or she is capable of tackling life's happy challenges.

excited delirium A condition in which patients have an increased sympathetic response and may become agitated, violent, combative, and paranoid; they may present with psychotic behaviors and may also have hallucinations, have an increase in strength, and become insensitive to pain or self-inflicted injuries.

hardware Solutions that take the form of computers, vehicles, tools, medications, or protective equipment.

high-reliability organizations (HROs) Organizations that operate in high-risk environments yet strive to maintain a learning atmosphere so as to minimize chances for error.

human perception time The time it takes a person to realize that he or she needs to react to an impending event.

human reaction time The time it takes for a person to react to an impending event.

humanware The people who are part of a team that has been directed to solve a particular problem.

incident command system (ICS) A management tool that helps people manage emergency incidents by identifying incident needs and setting priorities.

indirect costs The expenses and psychosocial effects related to the loss of functionality after injury, such as the inability to function normally at home, loss of ability to perform community services, and spousal/significant other adaptation to injury.

manual distractions Distractions that cause the emergency vehicle operator to take a hand off the ambulance wheel.

microsleep When the mind ceases to be aware of its surroundings and the eyes may close for a short period; it may last from a few seconds to a few minutes.

post-traumatic growth (PTG) An emerging field of study that demonstrates that survivors of trauma can actually grow and become "better people" through their willingness to build from traumas they have confronted.

postincident analysis (PIA) An activity involving team members that takes place after an incident response. It reviews performance of individuals and teams while focusing on learning lessons that can be applied to future incidents.

proprioception The reception and processing of sensory information that allows an individual to have an awareness of body position.

rate of closure The speed at which a vehicle overtakes another.

reactionary gap A formula that compares action to reaction, concluding that sudden action is faster than defensive action and that the closer a potential attacker is, the less time an EMS practitioner has to react.

safe patient movement behaviors Those actions selected by the EMS practitioner that minimize the risk of injury to patients, practitioners, and bystanders during patient movement events.

self-efficacy The belief that you are capable of performing in a certain way to achieve a certain goal.

sense making The ability or attempt to make sense of an ambiguous situation.

sensorimotor cues Sights, sounds, and smells that create an awareness of environmental conditions; this awareness may prompt a behavioral response.

siren syndrome When an emergency vehicle operator begins to drive aggressively and without regard for the conditions of the road during emergent operations.

situational awareness The state of being aware of what is happening to understand how information, events, and a person's actions will affect his or her goals and objectives, now and in the near future.

sleep debt The difference between the amount of sleep you get and the amount that your body needs.

software Solutions that take the form of rewriting training materials or procedures or developing checklists or policies.

stress Any event or situation that creates an emotional response.

surveying stance The body posture to take when defusing a stressful patient encounter. The body is slightly at an angle, with hands above the waist and out of the pockets, arms neutral, and knees slightly bent with the weight on the balls of the feet.

tapering A method to gradually direct traffic flow into an unaffected lane.

Traffic Incident Management (TIM) plan A preplanning document created with the input of all emergency responding agencies that ensures that all agencies will work together to secure the scene, maintain scene safety, care for and safely extract patients from the scene, and clear the scene as efficiently and safely as possible.

vehicle braking time The time it takes for the vehicle to stop.

vehicle reaction time The time between when the brake pedal is applied and when the brakes start working.

visual distractions Distractions that take the emergency vehicle operator's eyes off the road.

INDEX

Note: Page numbers followed by *f* or *t* indicate material in figures or tables respectively.

A

active shooter incidents, 69
advocacy, 18
AED. *See* automated external defibrillator
AEIOU-TIPS mnemonic, 76
aggressive driving, 26, 26*f*, 39
agitated delirium. *See* excited delirium syndrome
air ambulance, 47
airborne precautions, 104
alcohol hazards, 69
altered mental status, 72, 74
ambiguous statements/situations, 15
ambulance, 44, 97
    air, 47
    intended performance of, 97
    interdisciplinary approach to, 97
    internal structure of, 97
    safety issues for, 98
    stretchers, 62
American Council on Exercise (ACE), 89
anxiety, 85, 94
assessment "L" formation, 72, 72*f*, 81
assessment strategies, employing patient and environment, 56
automated external defibrillator (AED), 78
autonomic nervous system, 53

B

back injuries
    direct and indirect costs of, 55
    risks and consequences of, 54–55
bariatric patients, 53–54
bariatric stretchers, 63, 64*f*
Basic Life Support (BLS), 22
Battenburg pattern, 43, 43*f*
behavioral controls, 57
blood, 102
BLS. *See* Basic Life Support
BMI. *See* body mass index
bodies, 103
body mass index (BMI), 89, 90*f*
body positioning, 61
body substance isolation (BSI), 104

booby traps, 69
bowels, 102–103
breath, 102
BSI. *See* body substance isolation
bugs, 103
burnout, 88

C

cachectic, 57, 65
Candidate Physical Agility Test (CPAT), 5
carbapenem-resistant *Enterobacteriaceae* (CRE), 101
cardinal rule in conflict resolution, 18
cardiopulmonary resuscitation (CPR) seat configuration, 35
challenge, 18, 24
chevron pattern, 43, 43*f*
child restraint safety systems, 37
cleaning, 105–106
clinical assessment, 57
Clostridium difficile, 101, 102–103
Code Green Campaign, 87
codriving, 33–34
cognitive distractions, 33, 33*f*, 39
coherence, 18, 24
cold zone, 69
collective situational awareness, 10
collisions, avoiding, 26–31
    backing, 30–31
    data, 27
    personal experience, 28
    rate of closure, 31
    risk factors, 28–30
    speed, 31
combat distracted driving, 34, 34*t*
common driving distractions, 33
communicable disease, risks of, 101
communication, nonverbal, 71
complacency, 2, 8, 16
concealment, 74, 81
conflict resolution, 18–19, 24
conspicuity, 43, 49
contact precautions, 104
correctional facilities, 70, 70*f*
cover, 74, 81

CPR seat configuration. *See* cardiopulmonary resuscitation seat configuration
CRE. *See* carbapenem-resistant *Enterobacteriaceae*
crew resource management (CRM), 10, 13, 17, 24, 30
    communication loop, 19
    decision making, 20
    human error, reducing, 20–22
    humanware, 10–11
    incident command system (ICS), 11, 12*f*
    leaders, 13–14
    open communications, 17–19
    situational awareness, 14–17
    teamwork, 13
crime scenes, 68–69
    active shooter incidents, 69
    control zones, 69*f*
    hazards
        of alcohol, 69
        of illegal drugs, 69
CRM. *See* crew resource management
cumulative stress, 85

D

daily activities, movements performed by, 89, 91*f*
day-to-day stressors, 84
decision making, 19, 20
decision matrix, example of, 12*f*
defensive stance, 74, 75*f*, 81
Department of Transportation (DOT), 30, 46
depression, 85, 94
    reactive, 85
    trigger, 85
deranged, EMS practitioners violence, 73
desperate patients, 73
diabetic patient, 73
diet, healthy, 90–92
direct costs, 55, 65
discuss option phase, 19
disinfection, 105–106
distracted driving, 33*t*, 34
distractions, 30, 32–33
    dealing with, 16

distress, 84, 94
domestic violence, 73
DOT. *See* Department of Transportation
driving
    distractions, 33*t*
    texting while, 33
droplet precautions, 104
drugs, 72
    hazards of illegal, 69
drunk, EMS practitioners violence, 72
due regard, 31, 39

E

EMD program. *See* emergency medical
        dispatch program
emergency driving, 32
emergency lighting, 46
emergency medical dispatch (EMD) program,
        32
Emergency Vehicle Operator (EVOC) course,
        28
emergency vehicle operators, 15, 15*f*, 26,
        29–33, 35, 39
emergency vehicle safety
    avoiding collisions, 26–31
        backing, 30–31
        data, 27
        personal experience, 28
        rate of closure, 31
        risk factors, 28–30
        speed, 31
    codriving, 33–34
    distracted driving, 34
    distractions, 32–33
    emergency driving, 32
    helmets, 37, 37*f*
    patient compartment, 35–36
    preparation and ergonomics actions, 36
    risk mitigation, 36
    seat belt, 35
    total stopping distance, 31–32
    transporting patients, 37
    vehicle inspections and maintenance, 34–35
emergency vehicles, 28
    visibility of, 43
EMS practitioners
    assessment "L" formation, 72, 72*f*
    cover and concealment, 74
    crime scenes, 68–69
    defensive stance, 74, 75*f*
    delays in treatment, 77–78
    equipment failures, 78
    equipment maintenance, 64
    errors in patient care, 76–79
    excited delirium syndrome, 75–76
    exercise guidelines for, 89
    financial impact, 55
    fitness and health, 89–92, 89*f*
    goal of, 68

infections, 78–79
overview of, 68
patient falls, 77
patient/potential attacker, 73–74
physical and psychological harm to, 54–55
protection and safety of, 98
reactionary gap, 74, 75*f*
responsibilities, 78
restraint pitfalls by, 76
role of, 74
secure facilities, 70–71, 70*f*
situational awareness, 68
six Ds, 72–73
surveying stance, 72, 72*f*
unsafe environment for, 68
violence against, 72–74
weapons, 74
EMS Safety Foundation, 98
EMS Voluntary Event Notification Tool
        (EVENT), 28
EMS Workforce Committee, 98
energy sensor, 90
engineering controls, 58, 65
environmental assessment, 58
    lifting and moving plan, 59
environmental hazards, 54
equipment
    failures, preventing, 78
    lifting and moving, 62–64
errors in patient care, 76–79
    delays in treatment, 77–78
    equipment failures, 78
    infections, 78–79
    medication errors, 77
    patient falls, 77
eustress, 84, 94
EVENT. *See* EMS Voluntary Event
        Notification Tool
evidence-based practices, 56
EVOC course. *See* Emergency Vehicle
        Operator course
excited delirium syndrome, 68, 75–76, 81
exercise guidelines for EMS practitioners, 89
exhaustion, 88
exposure management, 105

F

fatal occupational injuries, 3, 3*t*
Federal Emergency Management Association
        (FEMA), 43
federal regulations, 98
FEMA. *See* Federal Emergency Management
        Association
First Response Resiliency Training, 86
fitness, 89–92
five Bs, 101–103, 102*t*
fixed physical obstructions, 58
frequent flyers, 77
friction-reducing devices, 62

G

geriatric patients, 54

H

hazards
    crime scenes
        of alcohol, 69
        of illegal drugs, 69
    environmental, 54
    to patient movement, 52
health, 89–92
Healthcare Infection Control Practices
        Advisory Committee (HICPAC) of
        Centers for Disease Control and
        Prevention, 104
healthy communication, 5
healthy diet, 90
    meal planning, 91–92
Heinrich's Law, 20
helmets, 37, 37*f*
HEPA respirator, 78, 78*f*
high-reliability organizations (HROs),
        10, 24
HIV. *See* human immunodeficiency virus
homeostasis, 84
homeostatic mechanisms, 3
hot zone, 69
HROs. *See* high-reliability organizations
human error, reducing, 20–22
human immunodeficiency virus (HIV), 102
human perception time, 32, 39
human reaction time, 32, 39
humanware, 10–11, 24
hydration in healthy diet, 90
hyperglycemia, 72

I

IAFC. *See* International Association of Fire
        Chiefs
ICS. *See* incident command system
in-house medical center, 70, 70*f*
incident command system (ICS), 11, 12, 23,
        24, 44
indirect costs, 55
infectious diseases, scene safety for
    cleaning and disinfection, 105–106
    communicable disease, risks of, 101
    exposure management, 105
    five Bs, 101–103, 102*t*
    personal responsibility, 101
    PPE, 103–104
    safety needle systems, 105
inquiry, open communications, 17–18, 17*f*
Institute of Medicine, 77
interdisciplinary approach, to ambulance, 97
International Association of Fire Chiefs
        (IAFC), 98
intersections, 28–29, 28*f*

K

kinetic energy of potential collision, 29

L

lateral transfer aids, 62
law enforcement, 44, 74, 76
leaders, 13–14
lift assist teams, 56
lifting, 56, 59–64, 60f
    body positioning, 61
    share the load, 60
line tapering, 45, 45f
literal translation, 52
long-term stressors, 84
lumbar sprain, 55

M

manual distractions, 32, 33f, 39
MDC. *See* mobile data computer
medication errors, 77
mental health, 84–85, 84f
methamphetamine (meth) lab, 69
methicillin-resistant *Staphylococcus aureus*
    (MRSA), 101
microsleep, 88, 88f, 94
mobile data computer (MDC), 32
moth effect, 46
motor vehicle crashes (MVCs), 3, 26–28, 68
    mobile communication devices, 33
movable physical obstructions, 58
moving plan, 59–64
MRSA. *See* methicillin-resistant
    Staphylococcus aureus
multi-lane intersections, 28
multi-vehicle responses, 29
MVCs. *See* motor vehicle crashes
myocardial oxygen consumption, 53

N

National Association of Emergency Medical
    Technicians (NAEMT), 26, 89, 98
National Highway Traffic Safety
    Administration (NHTSA), 3, 4, 31, 43
National Institute of Occupational Safety and
    Health (NIOSH), 55
necktie, EMS practitioners risk, 70
NHTSA. *See* National Highway Traffic Safety
    Administration
NIOSH. *See* National Institute of
    Occupational Safety and Health
nonemergent driving events, 4
nonverbal communication, 71
normalization of deviance, 78

O

obesity crisis, 89
observe and critique phase, 19

Occupational Safety & Health Administration
    (OSHA), 4
on-scene lighting modes, 46
open communications, 17–19
    environment, 11
open-mindedness, 99
Opticom device, 29, 46
optimal mental health, 84, 84f
OSHA. *See* Occupational Safety & Health
    Administration
out-of-service equipment, 64

P

PACE, 18, 18f
panacea, 97
patient care compartment, potential
    projectiles in, 35, 36f
patient care, errors in, 76–79
patient care report computers, 36, 36f
patient compartment, 35–36
patient handling, 52f, 55–57
    back injury, 54–55
    bariatric patients, 53–54
    behavioral controls, 57
    environmental assessment, 58
    equipment and device, 56
    equipment maintenance, 64
    geriatric patients, 54
    lifting and moving plan, 59
    patient assessment, 57–58
    pediatric patients, 53, 53f
    safe patient movement, 52–53
    unsafe, 53–55
patient/potential attacker, EMS practitioner
    violence, 73–74
patients
    altered mental status, 72, 74
    assessment, 57–58
    and environment assessment strategies, 56
    evaluation of, 57–58
    falls, 77
    lifting and moving plan, 59
    pediatric, 77
    physical and psychological harm to, 53–54
    restraint of, 76
pediatric challenges, transporting patients, 37
pediatric patient restraint system, 37
pediatric patients, 53, 53f, 63
    psychomotor skills with, 53
pediatric resuscitation tape, 77, 77f
personal health
    exercise guidelines, 89
    fitness and health, 89–92
    healthy diet, 90–92
    mental health, 84–85
    resiliency, 85–89
personal protective equipment (PPE), 103–104
    precautions, 104
personal responsibility, 5, 101

personal strategies, 21
physical examination of patient, 77
physical fitness, 89
PIA. *See* postincident analysis
pitfalls, restraint, 76
positional asphyxia, 76
post-traumatic growth (PTG), 88, 94
postincident analysis (PIA), 21–22, 24
posttraumatic stress disorder (PTSD), 86
powercots, 63, 63f
PPE. *See* personal protective equipment
practitioners, EMS
    assessment "L" formation, 72, 72f
    cover and concealment, 74
    crime scenes, 68–69, 69f
    defensive stance, 74, 75f
    delays in treatment, 77–78
    equipment failures, 78
    equipment maintenance, 64
    errors in patient care, 76–79
    excited delirium syndrome, 75–76
    exercise guidelines for, 89
    financial impact, 55
    fitness and health, 89–92, 89f
    goal of, 68
    infections, 78–79
    overview of, 68
    patient falls, 77
    patient/potential attacker, 73–74
    physical and psychological harm to, 54–55
    protection and safety of, 98
    reactionary gap, 74, 75f
    responsibilities, 78
    restraint pitfalls by, 76
    role of, 74
    secure facilities, 70–71, 70f
    situational awareness, 68
    six Ds, 72–73
    surveying stance, 72, 72
    unsafe environment for, 68
    violence against, 72–74
    weapons, 74
precautions, PPE, 104
prison, 70, 70f
proactive accident prevention, 5
proprioception, 54, 65
protocol based clinical judgment, 32
psychiatric issues, 73
psychological testing, 5
psychomotor skills, with pediatric patients, 53
PTG. *See* post-traumatic growth
PTSD. *See* posttraumatic stress disorder

R

rate of closure, 31, 39
reactionary gap, 74, 75f, 81
    aspect of, 68
    communication, 71
reactive depression, 85

refusal of medical attention (RMA), 22
relaxation, in resiliency toolbox, 88
resiliency, 85–89
   skills, 86, 86*t*
   toolbox, 86–89
      cognitive skills, 87
      goal setting, 86–87
      physical and behavioral skills, 87
      rest, relaxation, and sleep, 88
      social skills, 87–88
rest, in resiliency toolbox, 88
risk
   assessment, 20–21
   breaking down, 4–5
   identification and mitigation of, 5
   mitigation, 36
RMA. *See* refusal of medical attention
roadway operations, responsibilities in,
   42
   air ambulance, 47
   arrival and scene size-up, 44–46
   dangers of, 42–43
   emergency lighting, 46
   goal of, 46–47
   Traffic Incident Management Plans, 43
   vehicle visibility, 43–44
Rosenbaum, David, 16
"routine" lifting, 56

S

safe lifting techniques, 54
   body mechanics and training in, 55, 56
safe patient movement, 52–53, 56, 58
   behaviors, 57
safety, 3. *See also* practitioners, EMS
   EMS culture of, 97–99
   healthy communication, 5
   introduction, 2
   motor vehicle crashes, 3
   preplanning for, 43–44
   risk
      breaking down, 4
      identification and mitigation of, 5
safety needle systems, 105
scabies, 103

scene safety for infectious diseases
   cleaning and disinfection, 105–106
   communicable disease, risks of, 101
   exposure management, 105
   five Bs, 101–103, 102*t*
   personal responsibility, 101
   PPE, 103–104
   safety needle systems, 105
scene size-up, EMS, 68
seat belts, 27, 27*f*, 35
secure facilities, EMS practitioners, 70–71
   rules of response to, 71
   type of, 70, 70*f*
sedating medication, 88
self-efficacy, 87, 94
self-protective mechanism, 16
sense making, 18, 24
sensorimotor cues, 2, 8
siren syndrome, 31, 39
situational awareness, 10, 14, 24, 59, 68, 70
six Ds, EMS practitioners violence, 72–73
sleep debt, 88, 94
sleep deprivation on safety, impact of, 98
sleep, in resiliency toolbox, 88
   failure, 88
social support system, 87, 88
SOPs, 15*t*
staff, facility, 70
stair chair, 55, 55*f*, 63, 63*f*
standard precautions, 104
strenuous lifting, 55
stress, 84, 94
   communication skills, 71–72
   cumulative, 85
   deal with, 86
   signs and symptoms of, 86
stretchers, 58, 61
   ambulance, 62
   retention systems, 64
surveying stance, 72, 72*f*, 81
swerve alarms, 88

T

tapering, 44, 49
teamwork, 13

"The Effects of Sleep Deprivation on Fire
   Fighters and EMS Responders," 98
TIM plan. *See* Traffic Incident Management
   plan
total stopping distance, 31–32
traffic control, 45
Traffic Incident Management (TIM) plan,
   43, 49
training in safe lifting techniques, 56
transfer board, 63, 63*f*
transportation-related fatalities, 3*t*
transporting patients, emergency vehicle
   safety, 37
trauma shear, 70
trigger depression, 85

U

unsafe patient handling, 53–54
   bariatric patients, 53–54
   geriatric patients, 54
   pediatric patients, 53

V

vehicle braking time, 32
vehicle inspection, 34–35, 35*f*
vehicle maintenance, 34–35
vehicle reaction time, 32
vehicle speed, 29–30
vehicle visibility, 43–44
vehicles, respect your, 35
violence, EMS practitioners, 72–74
visual distractions, 32, 33*f*

W

warm zone, 69
water, 90
weapons, 74
worst case scenarios, 97

Z

zones of control, crime scene, 69, 69*f*